Who Moved My Curves?

4 Principles to Get Back Your Body and Mojo

Bernette Sherman

Mount Hope Media, LLC

Book Cover by Mount Hope Media, LLC

Print ISBN: 978-1-954636-13-2

To all the women trying to do more than just get by.
I see you.
I feel you.
I am you.
Together, we can thrive.

★★★

A special thanks to my husband, children, and my mother—without whom I wouldn't be the woman or person I am today.

Contents

Also by

Find Books at MountHopeMedia.com

Self-Help and Poetry

Love Me Journal (Self-love, Inner-child work)

Protect and Clear with the Divine (Spiritual clearing and protection)

Heaven is Now: Enough Excuses (Inspirational)

Resist Persist (Poetry)

Fiction

But First Crawl (Romantic Comedy)

Light of the Dark Moon (Fantasy)

Star Jumpers (Metaphysical Sci-fi)

The Story of Ervin James (Historical Fiction)

Out of the Woods (Fantasy)

Crossed (Paranormal light urban thriller)

Introduction

Dear Courageous Friend,

Choosing yourself isn't easy. In fact, it can be downright hard. But here you are, with this book and reading this letter from me to you. Dear friend, I believe you are courageous and I'm already rooting for you. That's right, out here in this great big world just know someone is believing in you and what you can do.

Like I told myself in the early days, there is always a day one. That means we can always start over, start fresh, and give ourselves another chance. You can do everything you dream of doing and create that body and the life you long to have. You don't have to wait until someday or when everything else is just right and perfect. Because that will never come.

Now is the time for you, your wellness, and your life. It's time right now to experience how it feels to be in a body that works with you and supports you. It's time to get your mojo back! Imagine that. Your life like you want it, sooner rather than later.

The four RENT principles I'll share with you in this book work extremely well, especially when you work them. Do them as I show you and you can transform your body and begin the transformation of your life for years to come.

I want the world for you. With all it's fun, joy, grandeur, and love. It's why I had to start here, with a book that begins with the body because it's where our minds and spirits reside. When we start here in the way I've shared with you, it is the beginning of limitless possibilities. Yes, I believe it. My next work will dive more deeply into rewriting our stories using the shero's journey framework and then manifestation. If you enjoy this book, please stick around and get on my email list so you don't miss those.

Grab the bonus resources, join my free group, and don't feel like you've got to do this on your own. As women we're better together. My friend, you will have days that are hard as that French bread that got left out in the open and other days that flow like a spring breeze. They're both ok. You're okay. You are worthy. You are deserving. You are divinely purposeful. You are loved. What you seek, you can have.

One more thing, when you've gone through this book and done the work, I'd love for you to let me know how it worked!

Love,

Bernette

P.S. Please leave a review at your favorite online retailer to help other midlife women get their body and mojo back as well.

P.P.S. You might also enjoy my romantic comedy, But First Crawl, available in paperback and as an eBook on Kindle and in KU.

Chapter One

Your Midlife Mojo

You've lived decades for this moment, through relationships, careers, disappointments, joys, and finding and re-finding yourself. You've felt success before, tasted victory.

Now it seems society wants to put you to the side, in favor of a younger model, forgetting that you carry the wisdom, experience, an inner power, and magic she, our world, desperately needs.

There's little time to connect with other women because life demands keep you busy, and you might even feel guilty about using those free moments you do have to spend on yourself. Unless it's for a nap because you're feeling drained.

If only this body of yours would act right. Doesn't she know you have things to do? A life to live? Being saddled with extra pounds, lower energy, mood swings, and for some of us, embarrassing hot flashes during key moments of the day and night sweats that steal much needed sleep, aren't helping.

The mirror and you haven't been on good terms lately. Did someone switch out your mirror for one from the fun house? I mean really! How else can you explain the fact that your curves moved? I mean who did that? Not just the shape of your hips, where your bottom now sits in your jeans, and that gravity hasn't done you any favors; but your curve of how you flow through life and move through your day.

Who moved your energy curve? Your mood curve and your heat curve? You've got spikes and valleys in all these areas now. There are so many curves that look nothing like they used to thanks to the midlife curveball trying to hit every single one.

And let's not even mention that the rest of the world has noticed it too. How do you know? You've gone invisible despite having more to offer to the world than you've ever had before. Can we mention the curve of your career and perceived value in the world? Where you were once on the top of the bell curve, you feel like you've fallen down the slope here too.

Surely, there's gotta be something better. Add to all this the creeping anxiety and a general sense of malaise that's settled in, and you hardly recognize yourself. Is there a single curve where it's supposed to be?

What happened? And, more importantly, how do you get back into the flow and get your curves working for you again?

If you're reading this book, that means you're in those middle years of life. You may be in your late thirties, forties, fifties, or even your early sixties. For some of us, we haven't hit the menopause window, but some of us have or are now on the other side. It can be a pretty wild ride in this midlife. With all this change, it's easy to lose the mojo we once had. It's easy to lose ourselves too, and feel like we've disappeared. But we don't have to settle for it and that's why you're here.

We can get back a new mojo and put our curves where they belong. This new mojo we create can support us during these midlife years and in menopause. I like to call these the freedom years and whether you've just opened the window, are crawling through it, or are on the other side there's a lot to look forward to.

You have the power to create mojo for your midlife that gives you the energy and vitality to live a healthy and vibrant life, for a long time.

Maybe you grabbed this book because I told you that you could get back your mojo without living in the gym, doing endless hours of hard cardio, or having to live a life of starvation. And I meant it.

The goal isn't to live in the gym. It isn't to run or do the elliptical machine or stair machine for hours and hours a week. It isn't to be on a restrictive diet until you hungrily take your last breath hoping it smells and tastes like chocolate ice cream or in my case, New York style cheesecake with cherries on top.

Instead, the goal is to live a balanced and vibrant life through midlife. It's to be healthy while enjoying your life.

How can you have your mojo if you can't go celebrate a friend's birthday or go on vacation and taste the foods that immerse you in the culture? Or just have a nice dinner out with family or your partner? Without choosing the salad…again. You deserve better.

And you can have it by mixing the principles I share in this book with a little magic. Maybe you don't call it magic, but it's definitely some manifestation happening!

You get to be in the flow of your divine feminine essence while using the four RENT principles and fairy dust (universal principles), I'll also sprinkle in to help you get back your mojo. When we use our mind, spirit, and body everything can be in alignment and it just flows better!

★★★

Before going any further, if you aren't into metaphysics, manifestation, or spirituality this book may not be for you. I want to tell you that in chapter one. I used to try to tone my magic and mojo down but I realized that this too is denying myself and once again putting myself as a non-priority. I told you, when you use these principles you get your mojo back – body and life. Once you have it, you won't want to dim it down or give it away again.

So, this is my one and only warning that if you don't like 'this stuff' put the book back, return it, or give it away, but don't be that person who leaves a bad review because it's the kind of book I said it is. It's a fitness and wellness and lifestyle book that uses practical lifestyle principles, mindset, manifestation, and universal laws. There, you have it.

You'll either love it, be unmoved by it, or be turned off. Whichever, I still want the best for you and hope you'll find the lane to walk in that lets you create your mojo for your epic life.

***

Everything your body needs is available to you. Your goals for your health and wellness are possible and whether you simply want to lose belly fat, get lean and toned, or lose significant weight–you can do it. You can feel better, be clearer, and more confident in your everyday life. You can get your body back, get your body snatched, or just have a body that functions better.

It's up to you. Completely. At the end of the day, there's only one person living inside your body so it should be one you love. It should be one that serves your goals and needs. It should be one that can carry you through living out your unique and divine purpose.

While this book does have information on menopause, it's not about menopause. There are other books on menopause out there. I know. I've read some. There are books written by doctors and scientists with all kinds of scientific information in them. These are great and helpful. Get them. Read them. I don't claim to be either a doctor or a scientist but I'll share a little science and research. I used to be a researcher in health policy and worked in community and public health programs.

There are tons of diet books and programs out there to help you lose weight, get skinny, get strong, eat a certain way and do it fast so you can look great at the reunion, on the beach, or for the holidays.

Who doesn't want that? Of course I want, and wanted, that too, but I wanted more.

Maybe you were just picking up a fitness book geared to us women going through the stress and changes of midlife and menopause. But what you'll get is more than that. You're getting a book that challenges you to look at how your lifestyle and mindset will help you get into a new place where you can thrive for life.

As a midlife woman in the menopause window, I know how important it is to feel good in our bodies. I wanted that for myself and I could've lost the excess weight using quick tricks and fad diets. I could've essentially starved my way into smaller jeans. But is that truly sustainable? Is it healthy? Would it have served my life and my values for the long-term? Would it have been the solution I needed? The answer to all those questions is no.

Without making different choices and adjusting our behaviors and mindset to line up with our bigger vision for ourselves and our lives, we just wind up going back to the old default settings and recreating what we were once comfortable with. We got used to the discomfort and that discomfort can fool us into thinking it's comfortable.

I couldn't fool myself any longer. I wasn't comfortable and I knew it. I refused to settle for a body that wasn't living up to my purpose. I couldn't live in my purpose when my body wasn't functioning like I needed it.

If you're in your forties, fifties, or sixties you probably feel like I felt before I said yes to treating myself like the divine feminine being I am. All of these decades give us shift after shift, but the truth is we do have a choice in how we shift. But with all the information out there today and our own body signals, we can be confused and overwhelmed about what to choose to then make the changes.

We can feel like our mojo has been stolen. And maybe it has. But like I said before, we can get it back.

That's why I've created this book to serve as a guide to get back your mojo during midlife. To help you create more wellness in your life and feel good. And do it without setting up a cot at your local gym, spending hours during torturous cardio, or surviving on boring salads and rice cakes. Even the idea that some of us think that's what we have to do for the rest of our lives makes me sad.

Because that way doesn't work at this age. It really never worked. And it's definitely not a recipe for getting your mojo back when you don't have the time or energy to make this season of your life more than beating the belly bulge, taking care of work, home, and managing whatever other daily surprises your body serves up.

You're here and are making time for you. So, it's important to keep yourself as a priority in your life and how you start this journey is key to whether you do that and for how long. That's why I'm sharing what I've coined the RENT principles, both practical and Universal principles, to live by.

These principles can not only help you ease some of your menopause symptoms, but help you get fit, stay fit, and thrive through midlife, living in your mojo, and being fit for the life you want. That's where it's at, friend! We can get out of the slump that seeps into every other area of our lives and finally feel good. Yes, love, both inside and out because this is about a lifestyle that supports your wellness.

My writing and work are generally geared to women because I believe that when women are healthy, whole, and happy our families, communities, and world will reflect that too. And when I speak to you, write to you, and support you, it's with that mindset. That you are the shero of your own epic adventure, even if you haven't truly stepped into your power. That shero is still in there, waiting to be revealed.

Getting your body and your life back is an amazing feeling, love. Believe me, your mojo is waiting for you. Your curves are ready to flow and move in alignment with who you are and what you desire. But before you dive into all the nuggets I'll share; do you know what you're after? Do you know why you actually want that mojo?

Midlife Mojo Vision and Goals

Getting my mojo back transformed my life. It started with getting my body back because that was the clearest sign that things weren't alright. In September 2023, I wanted to shed thirty pounds naturally by the end of the year. This would bring my BMI (body mass index) back to the top of the healthy range. I hadn't been there since my late thirties. It was an aggressive goal but I knew it was doable.

But it meant I'd have to commit. I'll share a little about my story in chapter three, but let's just say that I did commit. Otherwise, you wouldn't be reading this book by me.

Was it easy? No. Was it hard? Not really. Because I kept it top of mind that this was for me. This time, it wasn't for my kids or my family or my clients and would be clients or the spiritual community or aspiring writers or anyone else. It was only for me. I deserved it, and it would be worth it. I wasn't wrong.

If you want to make it work this time, you have to start here. Maybe you've tried diets, workout routines, and all the things before and it worked for a while. But then it failed. I know I did.

It can be frustrating and discouraging and honestly damaging to our bodies. But when you get it in your head that your health is the priority you'll shift how you approach your wellness journey.

That's what I want for you. As you start looking at the reasons you picked up this book, what you want to do and your goals, remember this time it really is about you.

You get to choose your midlife mojo goals. How will you feel? What will you do when you have your mojo back? If weight loss is a goal, what does that mean for you? If general fitness is a goal, what does that mean for you? Do you want to look better in your clothes, dance or play kickball, do active vacations and other activities, play with your friends, kids, or grandkids? All without panting and being afraid your blood pressure is getting too high?

Some of my goals, in addition to getting to a healthy BMI level, were to be able to do ten pushups and run one mile. Considering I couldn't do a single regular pushup and hadn't run a mile since college, these were big goals for me. Achievable, but big!

This book isn't focused on creating goals so I don't include that exercise here. I have a free four week workbook you can download through Ber netteSherman.com/midlifemojo, which includes the midlife mojo vision and goals questions along with questions from the RENT chapters of the book. You can print it out and use that journal as you read the book. I want you to be successful because it's finally about you, my friend. If you don't use the free workbook, before diving into this book, I suggest thinking and feeling through the following questions and writing them down somewhere you can refer back to.

Your Midlife Mojo Vision

1. Why is it important to you to get your mojo back, lose weight, or feel better?

2. How will you feel?

3. What will you be able to do differently?

4. What will change in your life?

Your Midlife Mojo Goals

1. What goals do you have for your health, fitness, and overall physical wellness?

2. How will you know you've reached those goals?

3. What milestones are there along the way to reaching your goal?

4. Can you write them down using the SMART method? Specific, measurable, achievable, relevant, and time-bound?

5. How will you recognize and reward yourself when you reach a milestone?

Keep your vision and goals somewhere prominent. You can write each goal on a sticky note and place them on your desk, bathroom mirror, or refrigerator. You can make them a screensaver on your phone or computer. You could put them in all these places so you are constantly reminded.

One tip for reaching your goals is to be mindful of them every single day. Revisit them, adjust them, write new ones down as needed. Whatever you do, look at them every single day to keep them top of mind.

Your vision and goals are for you alone.

You're saying to yourself that you are important enough to plan for and to set hopes for a future. And when you do that, you signal to the Universe that you're ready. And when we achieve our health and fitness goals, we get that extra boost to our self-esteem. We get to show ourselves that we are competent and able to do hard things and we get to improve our overall well-being at the same time.

My graduate degree was in policy analysis and evaluation and I spent years in program management in community and public health. One of the things we always did was set goals, milestones, and a plan to work backwards. What do you want to accomplish? By when? What resources do you need to be successful? What are you starting with?

Breaking down larger health and fitness goals into smaller, achievable steps can help you stay on track of your progress as you move towards milestones. When you reach a milestone decide how you'll recognize and reward yourself for the accomplishment, no matter how big or small it may seem.

By acknowledging you've reached smaller or major milestones you continue to build your confidence through competence and it reinforces positive behaviors and builds up your positive mindset. So many reasons to celebrate!

While you're celebrating, just remember not to do anything that'll set your progress back. Celebrating with a huge slice of chocolate cake and ice-cream after meeting your nutrition goals for the day, isn't celebration. Ignoring your walking goals for three days because you were consistent for one week isn't a reward for your progress. Celebrate in ways that affirm you, make you feel good, and support you in achieving what you've set out to do.

It'll be helpful for you to have practical ways to track your progress and a rewards system in place. This will help you pick out rewards that aren't subconscious attempts to sabotage you. Doing this ahead of time makes it easier to celebrate and stay committed to your journey.

I won't kid you, getting your mojo and your body back is gonna cost something. Time, energy, or money. Maybe all three. It took me three months, time in the gym, studying, and paying attention to my rest and nutrition, and money spent on a personal trainer. I also chose to invest in books and courses. You don't have to do all of that. In fact, you get to choose which of those three levers of time, energy, or money you'll pull.

Will there be sacrifice and compromise? Yes, there will be. But the more you follow the principles in this book the less these will feel like sacrifices and compromises. You'll see that you're making an investment in the only asset that is truly ever yours. Yourself.

And that's where this midlife mojo journey and magic begins. With you.

Chapter Two

Get Back Your Mojo

By the time we enter our middle years we're supposed to have it figured out. We know what we're doing and living the dream. Careers, family, relationships, and our health are humming along and we should be able to just coast along from now on.

Wait. Who ever said that was the deal? I would've signed up immediately and gladly signed the no return policy. That's right. Tell me it was going to be all good and I would be all in.

Then I turned forty.

There's nothing like a good plot twist!

I'd spent years as a writer and was sharing how I do world building at a writers' event held at a bookstore in August 2023. But something was missing.

And no, I couldn't have told you exactly what wasn't there.

It was like I had the idea for this epic story and I knew who the shero was supposed to be but I couldn't get past the middle.

She couldn't get past certain lessons successfully so she could move on to the next level. Something she wasn't able to recognize was holding her back. *She had a blind spot.* I had a blind spot.

Still I was in a situation where my health was going in the wrong direction, as it had over the past three years. I'd put on just over thirty pounds in that time.

This included my very own Covid-19 nineteen pounds, plus the additional weight from stress, being in perimenopause, and inactivity. And yes, of course, I knew I should have been exercising, but don't we all know that?

And suddenly I didn't know what I wanted to do with my life and little did I know that smack dab in the middle of this transitional decade, we would be hit with a global pandemic that would further rock my world. And probably yours too.

There I was, knowing the adventure I'd set out on was meant to be epic but I was thwarted at every turn. It was like a joke and everyone's laughing but you have no idea why.

I decided that even though I was still waiting to step into my epic life, it didn't have to look like the one I'd started writing. I changed the plot.

Sure, the end goal to have some positive impact on the world is still there, especially for women, but how I do it…that changed. I looked at the tools I held and remembered one very important thing I've built into every book I've written.

It's that you can't help others at the level of a shero until you first acknowledge your weaknesses, second, you choose to make those internal transformations, third, you train for that epic life, and fourth, you see the transformation on the outside as well.

Before I started my wellness journey in my late forties and through perimenopause, I felt like something was holding me back from really serving at the level my divine purpose has called me to serve. I'd been on a journey as a coach, healer, writer, parent, and partner. We'd had great success personally and financially. Our real estate ventures had done well, but something was missing.

It was only when I got my body back, or should I say, got back into my body, that I got the clarity and got in alignment so the Universe could deliver into me and through me.

Let's just say health is only one aspect. There's mindset, manifestation and money! Those other topics will be in future books and programs that are already in the works but your midlife mojo is a big enough topic by itself. So that's where we're starting.

The transformation is evident inside and out and the benefits go beyond my body to my entire life.

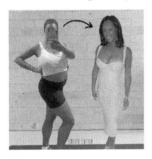

My friend, it's time to reclaim your mojo in this phase of your life. Time to reclaim your feminine power. It's time to ditch the naysayers saying it's impossible, too hard, or you'll just gain it back and know that you can do it and you can choose a different way for yourself. A way that brings in all of who you are physically, mentally, and spiritually. It's a way of wonder and wellness and that epic, mojo-filled life is here for you.

Chapter Three

Your Wellness Journey Awaits

If you're still reading this book that means you're pretty sure you want to make a change. Getting fit, losing that extra weight put on by stress and the changes in our body during midlife, including menopause, and feeling better are at the top of your list. You know it's time to set yourself up with the best chances for a long life in a body that feels good and functions like you want it to. And deep down, you know you're worth it.

If you're still on the fence about saying yes to yourself and what's possible, it's time to get off the fence, and step into the adventure that's calling you.

If you don't decide whether you're staying where you are or going for the vision and goals you wrote down in the first chapter, you may as well press pause right now. Why? The Universe will have a hard time knowing how to meet your desires and show up for you. And trust me, it's much easier when you are intentionally working with the Universal principles, rather than having them be in default mode.

Brave friend, this is your chance to write a new story for your life and what's possible. I wonder what new adventures might be waiting. You may be thinking. Yeah, I want to, but I don't know. It's so hard and what if I fail?

Change *is* hard. I know. And like I said before, it's okay. If it were easy, everyone would do it. Coaches and trainers and self-help books, like this one, wouldn't be needed. We'd decide to change and then just start applying the behaviors that support the change. But it doesn't usually work that way, because most people are only looking at behaviors and not using the magic with it.

I'm not going to go completely *wave your wand and click your heels three times and you'll have it* kind of magic on you. I'm a Capricorn and tend to keep at least one foot on the ground while reaching into the ethers. I'm going to tell you what I did, what I learned, what I've figured out can help and work for you, and how to apply Universal principles to be more successful, more quickly—without adding more stress on your body.

It's true that life during these middle years can be stressful enough, unforgiving, demanding, and seemingly unfair. I mean really, on top of everything else, we're also entering, in the midst of, or in the recent aftermath of menopause. And can we also ask why that wasn't a part of our sexual education classes? But I digress on that second point.

Menopause is technically the point in time when we've gone twelve months without menstruating, or having a period. Our bodies could go eleven months, we have a period, and then we don't bleed for six months, and have a period. If that's the case you're still in perimenopause. This book isn't just about menopause, but if you're a midlife woman, you'll be dealing with it or are dealing with it. That is if you haven't gotten past it already.

That's why I talk about a menopause phase or window, because all through this our hormones are just having their own party, and keep changing their minds about who's invited and then some are no-shows. It can be a hot mess!

It also leads to higher testosterone and cortisol levels and higher cortisol has a direct impact on how our body interacts with stress.

And it's that stress that can lead to how our bodies feel in these middle years. Oh joy!

The reality is that many of us are dealing with the effects of changing hormones on our bodies and we're seeing it clearly in our waistlines, feeling it emotionally, and dealing with it the best we can. I'm not judging. I'm just saying.

At the same time, we do have a public health crisis on our hands, that affects our economy and ability to continue to be competitive on a global landscape.

The obesity epidemic is real, and it can lead to other health conditions such as cardiovascular diseases, metabolic diseases, respiratory diseases, musculoskeletal disorders, cancer, and other conditions.

Poor health also impacts the workforce by putting a strain on businesses' healthcare costs. A workforce that requires more medical care is a more expensive workforce to cover and provide care for. Insurance companies end up increasing the employer's insurance rates and employers will pass that down by increasing their employees' insurance share. Some of the increased cost gets passed to consumers as well.

It pays to be healthier and to maintain a healthy lifestyle. It's why many employers offer wellness programs. A healthy workforce is more affordable and more productive. They'll also stick around longer because they're happier.

And if you're an entrepreneur or in a small business, this is even more important as healthcare and private insurance can be an even greater share of your revenue and costs.

The bottom line is that your health is impacting someone's bottom line, including yours. As I like to remind myself, *our health is our wealth.*

There is good news! Things can get better. Your body can feel good and your mind can feel like it's yours again. Isn't that worth raising a hand for?

I was pleasantly surprised that I not only managed to get rid of hot flashes and night sweats but my moodiness also softened. I can still be a little sharp-tongued and sarcastic since it's just in my Capricorn nature, but I was just being plain old short and snappy and it took my loving daughter to point it out.

Oh, and there was the brain fog and feeling like I couldn't find words when I needed them. I literally found myself hesitating to speak because the ideas were clear in my mind and then I'd open my mouth, and couldn't find the words. I admit, it scared me. I felt like I was sinking back into myself. Thankfully, I'm no longer afraid to speak and can flow off the cusp again.

When I took care of myself and put my health first, I got back my mojo and my wellness in every other area improved too.

It's a little magic mixed with mindset and science–all applied by you. That's powerful!

And, it's possible.

Without a body that can be in service to the mind and the spirit, all of the things you want to manifest and experience are going to be a lot harder to receive or achieve.

I'm here to help you get your body back and your mojo back so you can have that epic life, my friend.

The first step is to say yes.

Do you want this?

Will you say yes?

If your answer is yes, let's talk about the four RENT principles of Rest-Reset, Exercise, Nourishment, and Truth. And we'll talk about how you can apply these both practically and as simple Universal principles to get back your mojo in midlife.

The RENT principles will help guide you on your journey and are a way for you to continually check in with yourself. I'll also weave in Universal principles, like I said I would. In each chapter I'll briefly share the RENT principle as it can be applied as a Universal principle and then go into the meat of the chapter which is the RENT principle applied in fitness and wellness.

If you've ever heard of the principle 'as above, so below', think of that as an overarching principle. When you think of the RENT principles, there are the higher-level ones we apply spiritually and towards mindset and then the second level principles we apply physically, and often mentally. There can also be an overlap in the principles.

Throughout this book just remember that everything works together. The four RENT principles can change your body and your life.

Like I mentioned before my goal is to keep this book short enough to read and implement quickly. That means it's digestible but there will be a few portion sizes that are a bit larger, so take your time to chew on them thoroughly and mindfully, as that's how you'll feel more nourished and satisfied.

I've also included a four-week jumpstart guide in this book. The four-week free workbook is available with my bonus materials at BernetteSherman.com/midlifemojo.

Now, it's time to get into each of the RENT principles and experience what else is possible for your body and your life.

Chapter Four

Rest and Reset

The Western woman isn't doing so well. Our femininity has been wounded, we're stressed, depressed, unable to reset, and aren't getting enough sleep or downtime.

It's no wonder one in every five women in their forties and fifties is on antidepressants. Nearly one in every four over age sixty is. These are the highest rates of any group by age or gender!

I'm telling you, we as a group aren't okay and it's because we aren't able to slow down, rest and reset our minds, spirits, and bodies, and be genuinely supported. This is also why I made my group for midlife women. You can join it on Facebook. The link is available at BernetteSher man.com.

As women, we need to care for ourselves fully and in healthy ways. Love, if no one has told you this in a while, you matter. You matter.

Being in the divine feminine energy means being open to receiving. We can get trapped in the masculine energy of doing, giving, pushing, and striving to make changes happen in our lives when we need to allow change to happen.

It's amazing what we can do when we relax, get some rest, and let our energy reset and be receptive. Alot of Rs, I know. But it's true. Being in your divine feminine flow, especially starting with this first principle of rest and reset, will set you up for success with everything else.

Rest and Reset as a Universal Principle

In order to create through manifestation, we have to be in a mental space where we aren't subconsciously sabotaging ourselves with mind-fields laden with fear, insecurity, old stories, doubt, and unworthiness.

Rest and reset, as a universal principle, is achieved by creating energetic space for what you desire to manifest. It puts you in a space to receive. With fitness and wellness, rest is giving our body the chance to slow down, process, synthesize, regulate, and digest.

Spiritually, it's similar. Resetting allows you to clear out stagnant energy, undesirable beliefs, thoughts, and generally get rid of the waste taking up your energetic space.

When you slow down to clear out the mental and spiritual clutter there is space for what you really do want. I think of it like having to clear off my desk before I dive into a new project or make sure the dishes are all out of the sink and the counters are clear before I start cooking dinner.

It's hard to put something new and fresh into a place already filled with clutter or even things that aren't useful but taking up precious space. This is part of the law of attraction energy of being open to receiving.

As women, we are able to manifest more wellness, and everything else we want, when we create an inviting space to receive. It's why our creative center is our womb!

In this case you want to evaluate what's been holding you back so far from living a balanced and healthy lifestyle? It can be almost anything, but you have to start digging into what it might be, so you can pull it out. Once it's out you've got space to plant new ideas and let new behaviors take root.

For example, I had tried for years to shed excess pounds but I couldn't seem to get them off of me. It had only been a few extra pounds at first, less than ten. Then, it crept up when the menopause window cracked open. I had to rest and reset, using meditation and self-reflection, to process my reasons for holding onto the weight.

I had my reasons but after some forgiveness work and self-love work done using the haiku poems in my *Love Me* journal, I was able to do what I needed with those stagnant stories keeping me and my mojo separated. Once I purged the old stories, I could rewrite my stories and have space for the new version of the shero I wanted to be.

What stories are you telling yourself about your overall health and wellness? Are there stories that certain health conditions just run in your family, such as diabetes or high blood pressure? Are there stories of things you say you're not good at? Like you aren't good at dancing or planning ahead.

Do you have stories about what you don't like, such as green vegetables or lean meats? Perhaps you're telling yourself that you never could lose ten pounds in a month without doing unsustainable things? Maybe you tell yourself that other people have that body or can look a certain way, but not you.

Go through memories for anything around how you judge how you look, how you feel about your body and size. Go through memories about your relationship with food.

Dig into the memories that affect *how* you eat. For example, were you often rushed or felt like you'd miss out if you didn't hurry and eat so you could get seconds?

What about your memories that impact *when* you eat? Were mealtimes random, late, or unreliable? Were you always very hungry by the time you were fed?

What about *where* you eat? Were you eating in the car, while on errands, or otherwise on the go?

Even consider what might connect with why you eat. These may not necessarily be specific memories, but feelings that trigger a behavior. For example, do you eat when you're hungry and seeking nourishment, or do you eat when you're feeling bored, anxious, restless, sad, numb, or depressed?

Write it all down. Don't skip a memory if it comes up, especially if there's still emotion tied to it. These stored memories might be impacting you right now and the evidence could be in how you feel about your body, treat your body, and the relationship you have with food.

What if you could use the rest and reset principle here to bring up this belief, memory, or nonbeneficial feeling around your body and eating and purge it? You could then replace it with something that will actually serve you and that divine purpose you're here for. Wouldn't that be wonderful?

Part of rest and reset is forgiving those old stories we hold and whatever helped create those stories in the first place. Just like in other coaching I do, especially around abundance, wealth, and prosperity, there are plenty of stories that affect our bodies and what we hold in our bodies.

However, there are also a lot of tools we can use to reset our stories, but forgiveness is one of the simplest tools, even if it doesn't always feel easy. I also use some other tools, including somatics, for releasing stuck stories and energy.

But for now, we'll keep it simple so you can get on with getting your mojo back. With this forgiveness tool, you can't really get it wrong when you do it with the right intention. You can do it anywhere and don't need any extra tools besides yourself.

There is a Hawaiian practice for forgiveness and reconciliation called ho'oponopono. While it is traditionally practiced as a ritual and has a specific process to follow, you can benefit from using some of the elements. I use just the four phrases to clear and forgive beliefs, patterns, and blocks that don't serve my highest good.

The thing is, sometimes stories, beliefs, patterns, and blocks are intricately layered. You clear one level and think you're fine until you find yourself at a plateau and then have to clear and forgive something else.

It can be very closely related to what you've already cleared but it's deeper so you didn't know it was there until you removed the other layer. It doesn't mean the clearing isn't working if you have to clear something again or at a deeper level.

The four phrases you can use as part of with ho'oponopono are:

- I'm sorry.

- (Please) forgive me.

- Thank you.

- I love you.

Can you say these in a different order? Yes. You can even give forgiveness to someone else. Even when you do this, you benefit. Forgiveness given to someone else is also forgiveness for yourself.

This is about the intention to clear and remove blocks. You can't get this wrong, when your intentions are right. You may have to repeat the phrases multiple times and when something comes back up while you're still working on clearing the blocks and limiting beliefs around your health and wellness, just do it again. You can also say the phrases while moving your body as in the exercise section. This compounds the clearing of energy.

Once you feel the energetic release of that block, it needs to be filled. Nature doesn't like a vacuum, or any empty space, and it seeks to fill it!

What new wellness story will you tell yourself in place of the old one? Write that down somewhere and hold on to it. You may even want to write it as an affirmation. If you need a little help, here's an affirmation you can try.

This is an important step if you want to manifest that body and your mojo. It can feel uncomfortable and you might want to stop. and clear it in the Rest and Reset step.

As with anything else you pay rent on, if you want to keep the gains, you have to keep up the payments. In this case, you may have to come back and do some more clearing.

When you do this exercise, you can energetically begin to shed the extra weight of old beliefs, stored memories, and feelings you've been carrying and no longer need to. It's okay to let them go.

***

Rest and Reset for Wellness and Fitness

A good night's sleep. It sounds so easy. But too many of us don't get the sleep we need, especially on a daily basis. The result? We have a bunch of people who are tired, worn out, and wind up cranky, irritable, and low on patience.

Add to that the other hormonal changes and it's pretty much a recipe for nightmares. If you were getting enough sleep to have them! Suffice it to say, rest is something we need and aren't getting enough of.

No wonder we're feeling the pressure from everyday stress and unusual stress even more than we might normally. Rest is a crucial part of stress management.

Watching your RENT starts with rest and reset because this can be a main culprit for everything else we experience in our bodies, especially during the perimenopausal and menopausal years.

Most of us think that getting more rest and relaxation means sleeping and vacationing but it's so much more than that.

The changes brought on by midlife and the added stress that perimenopause, menopause, post-menopause put on our female reproductive cycle are a major cause for increased cortisol and metabolic disorder.

If you suddenly found yourself with a pooch in your forties, it's not just you, love. Add regular life to this such as family, relationships, finances, careers, and other stressors and it's a recipe for the battle of the belly bulge. Like many other women, I found myself on the losing end.

While the actual reduction of stress is outside the scope of what I can provide you with here, I hope what I share can help you respond better to stress.

Improve Your Stress Response

We're supposed to not just live, but thrive. Yet chronic stress is straight up killing us! Heart disease is the number one killer of women in the United States and a whopping eighty percent of us reading this book (between 40 and 60) have at least one risk factor for coronary heart disease.

What's going on with us isn't working. Between the depression and depression medication and heart disease, clearly, we have gotten out of our nurturing and feminine flow. And it would be insane to keep doing the same thing that isn't working and has gotten us into the frazzled state we're in.

It's time to let your feminine energy flow as it was meant to. Being stuck in the masculine way of doing things has gotten many of us into this situation and it's not going to get us out of it.

To help rebalance your system, try techniques like meditation or deep breathing to activate the parasympathetic response. Regular exercise, getting enough sleep, and eating a healthy diet can also help.

Remember, finding what works best for you takes time, so don't get discouraged if you don't see results right away.

This book will cover exercise and nutrition as part of the RENT principles so in this chapter we're going to talk about improving our rest and how we reset.

Now, most of us think about metabolism as having to do with how much we're eating. At the same time, most of us noticed that around thirty to thirty-five we just couldn't eat like we used to. That's because metabolism isn't only about calories in and calories out. It's metabolic and is impacted by other hormones and stress.

Our bodies have a complex system called the autonomic nervous system (ANS) made up of two main parts called the sympathetic and parasympathetic systems.

These two systems work together to maintain balance, or homeostasis. Our fast-paced lives mean that many women are chronically stressed and this leads to our sympathetic nervous system being called on more than it should and our cortisol levels increasing and often staying elevated.

I don't want to overwhelm you with tactics to get to a state of better rest. I want to offer you a few tools you can use along with the exercise and nutrition that will be in the following chapters.

Let me also mention the last principle of RENT which is Truth. Following your truth in whatever you do is more important than what I or anyone else tells you. Always check in with yourself, your body, your mind, and your spirit when taking action so that what you do is both inspired and intentional.

So while I'll talk more about being in alignment with our truth later, I want to mention it before I share these practices to help you create ease and regulate your autonomic nervous system.

When we're feeling stressed, we need to tell our body it's going to be alright and to treat her gently and lovingly. There are a few ways to shortcut the time it takes to get back to homeostasis by how we respond to stress.

Mindfulness

Mindfulness techniques, such as meditation and deep breathing, can help reduce stress levels by activating the parasympathetic nervous system.

In a recent review of literature on the impact of mindfulness-based stress reduction (MBSR) on healthcare professionals, it showed that MBSR was effective in "reducing HCPs experiences of anxiety, depression and stress. MBSR was also found to be effective in increasing HCP levels of mindfulness and self-compassion."

As midlife women we can experience increased anxiety as an effect of hormonal changes and mindfulness-based interventions can have a moderate, but positive, effect on anxiety.

A literature review of a dozen studies showed mindfulness interventions to be as effective as cognitive behavioral therapy in reducing anxiety (Fumero, et al 2020) .

We can practice mindfulness in many ways but the important thing is to find something that feels right for you and that you can practice easily and regularly.

Here are three ways you can practice mindfulness without having to make major adjustments to your life (because you don't need to add that stress). I'll share techniques for each one so you can practice.

- **Breathwork:** Breathing brings us to the present and can activate the parasympathetic nervous system.

- **Body scan:** Brings our attention inward to notice in ourselves, without judgment, and keeps you in the present.

- **Walking:** Helps to activate EMDR naturally and reduce stress, while we notice what's happening around us. We can also be mindful by paying attention to our senses as you walk: the feel of the ground, the sounds around you, the temperature of the air.

Breathwork

The Physiological Sigh

I love this tool because it doesn't require any special skills, training, equipment, or place to do it. Wherever you are, you have your breath.

You've probably already done this without knowing it and if you're in my generation, you probably got the side eye from a parent or teacher for doing it. Many of us were taught to not to huff or even breathe too loudly when we were frustrated.

What they, and I didn't know, was that this act of huffing was actually our body's natural attempt to regulate and get back into a parasympathetic state. By holding our deeper breath and trying not to offend, we were actively working against ourselves.

Just like slow breathing can work, this sigh works, and quickly. Yes, I've tried it out and tuned into my body (another practice shared below) to see how I felt after doing the physiological sigh, which is also called the cyclic sigh.

It's fairly simple with a focus on the importance of the double inhale. If you've ever taken care of a baby or seen them falling asleep you may remember this subtle double inhale as they drifted off. It's like their little bodies know to put themselves into this peaceful state.

Somewhere deep inside we all hold this wisdom, it's just been pushed down for many of us because, especially as women, we weren't supposed to show our frustration - even by sighing too heavily.

But the sigh has power!

According to Nicole Vignola in the book Rewire, this double inhale serves to open up the deflated alveoli. When this happens it allows more oxygen to be taken in by the area surface of our lungs.

In Rewire she says it's one of the most effective ways to bring us back into a parasympathetic state. This is why it's first the first practice in the list.

How to do the physiological sigh?

To do this cyclic sigh you'll take two quick but deep breaths in through your nose, hold for a second or two, and then exhale slowly through your mouth. Then you repeat as your body relaxes and calms, dissipating the stress with each inhale and exhale.

Physiological Sigh Instructions

Two quick and deep breaths through the nose
Hold for a second or two
Exhale slowly through the mouth
Repeat as needed

Deep Breathing

Breathing is a mindfulness technique and helps us activate the parasympathetic nervous system because it brings us into our bodies and the present. When we're paying attention to the breath it's difficult to pay attention to anything else. It's why some meditating practices solely focus on breathing as a way to bring relaxation.

Another method of breathing is to breathe deeply in through your nose (if possible) and out through your mouth. Imagine the breath moving through your body or into the space where you feel stress, then hold your breath for several seconds, before you release it slowly. If you can do a count of five to inhale, hold for five, and exhale for five this is a great start.

Deep Breathing Instructions

Take a deep breath for a count of five in through your nose
Hold for a count of five
Exhale for a count of five through your mouth

The Body Scan

This mindfulness technique can be done in as little as a few seconds or you can do it for longer, allowing yourself to fully immerse yourself in a restful experience and settle into a parasympathetic state.

The body scan technique asks you to pay attention to your body and its sensations. For some of us this is going to be uncomfortable. For many reasons, we don't wish to feel our bodies because we've become disconnected due to things that may have happened in the past and stories and traumas we hold.

If this feels like too much for you, acknowledge your present truth, without judgment, and do something that brings you ease and joy.

If you want to try the body scan you can sit or stand and then bring your awareness to the top of your head and pay attention to the sensations and feelings that come up.

For this exercise, you aren't judging them, you're only noticing them before moving down through your head, shoulders, chest, arms, stomach, abdomen, legs, and your feet. If you are familiar with your chakras, you can also follow those and then move down to your legs.

The idea is to bring your awareness back to you, the present moment, and a connection to yourself.

Body Scan Instructions
Sit or stand in a relaxed position
Bring your awareness to the top of your head
Notice any sensations and feelings, without judgment
Continue scanning from top of head to toes

Walking

Walking is definitely a feminine power move. Not in an *only women walk* type of way but in a *it's in our DNA* type of way.

Our female ancestors were gatherers, walking miles to forage, usually in community. Our bodies are made for this slow, leisurely movement that is a relaxing source of exercise.

When we are walking for mindfulness, we add the benefit of stress reduction. Mindful walking adds intentional noticing of our surroundings and the sensations we experience.

You'll pay attention to the sounds around you from the rush of wind to a babbling brook or birds and insects. You'll notice your environment with the other senses as well for sights and smells. You may even use touch by feeling the softness of a leaf or the rough texture of bark.

The idea is to be fully present in your surroundings. When we do this, we also get a sense of our connection with the world and with nature.

Another proven benefit of walking is something called EMDR or Eye Movement Desensitization and Reprocessing. This is a relatively newer form of psychotherapy often used to treat trauma and post-traumatic stress disorder.

I won't get into EMDR here, but the process of walking and noticing and the rapid eye movement that occurs when walking in nature has a very similar effect on us that EMDR in a clinical setting has, according to Bessel A. van der Kolk, in his book The Body Keeps the Score.

Walking is one of the most amazing, and possibly underrated, tools for us. I'll talk a little more about walking in the chapter on Exercise to share how to walk as a midlife woman, especially if you are in menopause, so it's a way of exercising and doesn't add stress.

Rest, Reset, and Relaxation

Our changing hormones can result in restless nights. Maybe you've noticed more bathroom breaks or night sweats. Those changing hormone levels mean less estrogen and that means our serotonin levels drop too.

And then through a series of chemical reactions our body occasionally gets this signal that we're running hot. When this happens it sends blood surging to our skin so we can cool back down. Enter the hot flash.

These surges can happen at night too, causing night sweats that wake you up.

So in this section I'll give you some tools and techniques for getting more rest, relaxing, and recovering from stress-inducing activities, like exercise.

Sleep and Relaxation

Sleepless and restless nights will catch up with the best of us and faster than we think. Surviving solely on caffeine and sugar is not the answer, but caffeine isn't all bad. It's just not the answer to a chronic lack of sleep.

If we're also in perimenopause and menopause our body is like a preadolescent or adolescent. We're going through all these changes and mood swings while our body tries to figure out who it wants to be next. For those of you who haven't hit this yet, doing the work in this book can help you have a better experience. I don't believe we have to claim our mother's experiences as our own. You get to write your own midlife story.

And can't we write some stories? Our minds and imaginations are so active. It can be helpful if you're trying to be creative but not so much when it's stories of doom. Like I mentioned before, anxiety, which can lead to depression, is a common problem in midlife. Our minds are busy (hence the prior mindfulness techniques) and our bodies are trying to regulate, sometimes waking us up or making it hard to relax and fall asleep.

You might feel like a hot mess. And whether it's from changing hormones or just being in this phase of life, you're not alone and there is hope.

If you have trouble getting to sleep, having a sleep routine and preparing your environment to sleep are important. These two things can help you get to sleep and to get back to sleep if you wake up. Let's talk about them.

Sleep Environment

How relaxing is your bedroom? Does your sleeping area give you a sense of calm and peace or does it stimulate you? A messy or disordered room can excite the mind and even lead to more stress, kicking off other subconscious feelings of disorder and chaos. Your bedroom shouldn't make you feel on edge. Definitely not something you need while trying to sleep.

Consider making your bedroom a place of peace. If it's neat and orderly but you can't relax in there, consider burning some sage to clear the energy in the room.

You might try adding battery-operated candles or lamps with dimmers to create a more relaxing ambience. If it's helpful to have sleep music, consider having a sound machine or even a Bluetooth enabled sleep headband. I have one of these and I swear by it, especially since my lovely husband sometimes snores and that isn't so lovely.

Sleep Routines

Have a bedtime routine to train your body and your brain. Perhaps a non-stimulant tea, hot bath with Epsom salts, and massaging lotion into your skin is part of the process.

The idea is to do activities that calm you rather than energize you. You may want to start your bedtime routine at least thirty minutes beforehand. If a bath is part of the routine, you may have to start that sooner to have enough time to relax without feeling rushed.

We can also have trouble getting into a parasympathetic state in the evening because we haven't begun to unwind.

If you scroll social media or read news on your phone before bed and find yourself unable to get to sleep for a while after this, try shutting your phone off entirely thirty minutes before you want to get to sleep.

Read a physical book or perhaps use a dedicated paper-white reader. You can even read by candle light or use an artificial candle with low light output.

The light receptors from screens tell us to be alert, and keep us up. Just like in the morning you want to open the blinds to let the light in to wake you up for the day, removing excess light will help in the evening.

Part of your sleep routine could include setting up your environment to support healthier sleep habits.

Relaxation for Sleep

In addition to having sound sleep habits and a relaxing environment you may need to get your body into a parasympathetic state after your mind and spirit have started to unwind. Our bodies hold stress and tension but we can release a lot of it with muscle relaxation.

The following natural techniques can help you relax and prepare for sleep.

<u>Contrast Hydrotherapy:</u> For contrast hydrotherapy *you'll a*lternate between hot and cold water. For

example, take a hot bath and then jump into the hot shower or vice versa.

If trying to get to sleep, finish on hot since your body will naturally try to cool down. If you do try contrast hydrotherapy, do it one to two hours before bedtime but don't do a stimulating activity afterwards.

Progressive Muscle Relaxation: For progressive muscle relaxation, slowly tense your muscles starting in your feet and hold for several seconds and then relax, working your way up your body until you feel the tension release. So you will tense, hold, relax. Tense, hold relax. Once you're done you can repeat the process as you need. It's very effective.

General Relaxation and Recovery

While the two above techniques for relaxing are appropriate for getting ready for sleep, you may not want to go to sleep and instead you may just want to relax and take some stress off. For example, you've got something important to do, like a presentation or athletic endeavor, and you're feeling a little anxious. In this case sleep is not the goal.

The below activities with an asterisk can also be excellent for post workout recovery or recovery after doing something strenuous or particularly stressful. Maybe you do one before that presentation and another after!

This is not a comprehensive list but these activities can help you relax before bed and in general:

- Spending time with pets as long as they aren't stressing you out

- Cuddling

- Meditation

- Spa treatments*

- Leisurely walking, especially in nature*

- Drinking herbal teas

- Napping

- Sitting in nature

- Reading

- Creative activities

- Listening to classical or spa music

- Sauna therapy*

- Restorative and yin yoga*

- Stretching and foam rolling*

To regulate stress and promote overall well-being during this transitional period, we can try different activities to see what feels right for us. In addition to everything I've already mentioned regular physical activity also contributes to stress management.

Stress management is an ongoing process, like most things we do for our health and wellness. Finding what works best for you might mean having to experiment with some of the techniques here or others you discover. If you don't like something, that's fine. There are multiple options and you get to choose what you like and what you can stick with.

Now, let's talk about adding more joy to our lives to support our wellness and increase hormones that make us feel good, like dopamine, serotonin, oxytocin, and endorphins.

More Ease and Joy

When I started my wellness journey, aside from hitting the gym and changing my nutrition and diet, I decided that I had to have more ease and joy in my life. This became a non-negotiable for me. If stress and trying to be what I thought the world wanted or expected me to be had put me in this condition, I knew it wasn't going to be the answer for how I got out of it.

What was my divine feminine yearning for? I wanted to be more in touch with that feminine and yin energy. I had to be in order to break through the overactive sympathetic nervous system and heal the effects of the changes happening in with my hormone and chemical balance brought on by changes in my reproductive hormones.

I had to step into my feminine energy, which is an energy of receiving, nurturing, and harmony. How could I do that? What did that even mean?

It meant finding more ease in my life and doing things that brought me joy. Your ease and joy will be unique to you but you need to explore that for yourself. When we know how to get into a state of ease and a state of joy we can move out of a state of unhealthy stress.

If you've followed me or my journey you may have seen that I am seeking to create an EPIC life with more wellness, joy, love and abundance. That joy part is important. When I started this chapter I told you that having more ease and more joy were key to my transformation.

When you've experienced prolonged stress or chronic stress it may feel hard to get back into a parasympathetic state, but I hope you'll try the above techniques to train your body and your brain how to regulate and be in homeostasis, that state of balance.

Finding your joy will help.

I fell in love with taking care of myself–body, mind, and spirit.

I also freed myself from the self-imposed beliefs I had around who I was supposed to be and what I was supposed to do in order to satisfy my ideas around external expectations of me.

I had to let it go.

Why?

It was stealing my joy and I knew it. I felt drained when I thought about doing activities associated with it. Now, I have the energy to do that work again, in a different way. I now have a very clear focus and intention with that work because it's no longer isolated but part of my bigger mission surrounding how I serve and support other women.

Finding your joy doesn't have to be difficult. It might mean doing some of those previous relaxation or mindfulness techniques and then tuning into your inner self and possibly your inner child. What lights you up? I love dancing, singing, theater, and movies. I love to travel, and be with my family.

I love to write, even if the marketing and publishing part aren't so much fun. But these things bring me joy. I also love to be of service, but when I was in the midst of healing myself, I couldn't be of service to anyone else except myself.

I don't think joy has to be completely separated from wellness, love, and abundance. We can find joy in creating a lifestyle of wellness. We can find joy in self-love, loving our children, family, partners, careers, and in our creativity.

How can we experience more joy in those areas? We can even find joy in creating abundance and wealth when we bring back the divine feminine way of nurturing and being in community.

Wouldn't it be more fun to build wellness and wealth by taking a page out of the men's handbook? They mix business and pleasure all of the time. We can do that too while also nurturing each other, ourselves, and creating community and not just deals.

What brings you joy? Here's a few ideas to help you get brainstorming.

After getting into a relaxed state, let yourself be present with each idea and see how it feels in your body. With this list, think about specific things you might do under each bullet. A more detailed list is available in the resources accessible through Bern etteSherman.com/midlifemojo. When you consider the item, do you feel light, heavy, excited, anxious, nervous, get the chills, want to squeal, or run away? You might even feel excited and then get nervous about something. It's okay. Notice the sensation and make a note of it. Come back and revisit the things that gave you a sense of positive excitement and repeat the exercise.

Joy List

- Spending time in nature

- Creative pursuits

- Physical activity

- Lifelong learning

- Service to others

- Connecting with loved ones

- Travel and exploration

- Mindfulness practices:

- Hobbies

- Music

- Cooking or baking

- Caring for pets

- Playing with children

- Enjoying entertainment

What brings you joy? I hope you've come up with a few things that bring you joy and can lift your mood.

Be Supported

If you find that you cannot manage your stress or are experiencing anxiety or depression that doesn't allow you to function normally or is not normal for you, please seek professional support.

We deserve to be supported. As we allow ourselves to be in the divine feminine energy, we realize that means allowing ourselves to receive. Receiving includes being open to getting the things we need to thrive.

Finding time to nurture ourselves, rest, reset, and recover will always be a challenge when we have other competing other demands. But what if we could start putting our needs on the front burner with the principle of the power of one and five?

The Power of One in Rest and Reset

The power of one principle can be applied in a few ways. You can choose to do one thing. You can do one thing for one minute. You can do something once. If you do one thing, you might choose to do that one thing again. You can do something for one minute or do it one time. You're already there, how about one more? Again?

There are many activities in the above lists. Choose one thing to do for just one minute. Perhaps it's sitting in silence for a minute or doing the deep breathing for a minute? It may be choosing to read one thing positive or inspirational such as a poem, something from a book, or from someone you follow online.

The idea is to start, experience it, grow from it, and try it again.

What if you applied the power of one every day? Try picking one thing you'll do to support yourself and reduce your stress or improve how you rest and recover.

The Power of Five in Rest and Reset

The power of five takes it another step by having you show up for yourself for a longer, but very doable, timeframe. Perhaps you take five minutes to plan out how you'll build a consistent sleep routine into your life. Maybe it's a five-minute meditation, hot shower, or listening to relaxing music.

It may even be taking five minutes to clean up your space so you can relax. A five-minute walk in nature can do wonders for your mood and stress levels. In the grand scheme of things five minutes isn't long and we can all find five minutes, if we want to.

Midlife Mojo Habit Maker

- What has been your biggest challenge with getting the right amount of rest, reset, and recovery time?

- What has been your biggest challenge adding more opportunities to experience ease and joy?

- What one thing could you do today to begin shifting how you rest, reset and recover? Try picking one thing from the lists above. Can you apply the power of one or five?

- What one thing could you do today to begin increasing opportunities to experience joy? Try picking one thing from the lists above. Can you apply the power of one or five?

- What one thing can you do in the next week to continue supporting your rest, reset, and recovery needs? This could be establishing a new sleep routine, building in time for a recovery activity, or having a talk with your family about your goals and how they can support you.

- What one thing can you do in the next week to continue support having more joy?

Rest and Reset Wrap Up

- What's one thing you learned from this section?

- What one thing stood out the most to you in the Rent section?

- What one thing do you always want to remember?

Affirmations

- *I clear the beliefs and stories I no longer need and know that I am worthy of a body that serves me and my divine purpose.*

- *I am easily able to bring my body, mind and spirit to a state of rest and peace.*

- *My life is filled with ease and joy.*

Chapter Five

Exercise

Having a life we love, especially as we get older and have more responsibilities, requires that we exercise our power to take inspired and intentional action. According to Dictionary.com one of the definitions of exercise is "to put (faculties, rights, etc.) into action, practice, or use".

Exercise is all about movement and action. It's putting energy into motion. We have physical exercises we do, mental exercises, and spiritual exercises. Usually the goal is to bring something into better practice or conditioning.

We can easily see how this applies when we think about physical exercise. Our bodies get stronger, leaner, and we get in better shape (condition).

Before we exercise our body, it can be helpful to align this principle with mind and spirit as well. As you know, everything is connected.

Exercise as a Universal Principle

We're going to put into practice the use of inspired action to manifest the body we want more quickly. Pair this with physical exercise and you'll be astounded at how the weight you've been carrying is lifted off of you.

When it comes to our spiritual, mental, and physical practices we can't leave the outcome or the process to whim and chance. Being intentional means we also have to believe certain things about ourselves and what's possible.

We need inspiration aligned with who we are and what we desire for ourselves. Otherwise we won't build intentional, healthy, and practical life or lifestyle habits and will instead fall for quick fixes or just feel like it's hopeless.

This is true whether you're building a skill to use in your career, to improve the quality of your life, for fun, or for your health.

Applying this as a universal principle means truly getting into alignment with our full selves. You don't create a body you love and that serves your needs in a vacuum.

The Key Steps for Inspired Intentional Action

1. Get inspired.

2. Decide on the inspired actions to take.

3. Be intentional by planning around those inspired actions (don't leave to whims and chance).

4. Repeat.

Is this simple? Absolutely.
Is it easy? Not necessarily.
Is it doable? Yes!
Will you execute it perfectly? Not likely.

And that's okay. It's about progress and consistency and not perfection. Give yourself the grace and space to try things, see what you are capable of, fail, adjust, and go again. That's what we do. That's what people who choose to live epic lives do.

In three months I naturally shed thirty-two of those extra pounds I'd put on and got stronger using exercise, nutrition, mindset, and lifestyle principles. I went in HOPING it was possible, began the journey and started BELIEVING it was possible, and came out the other side KNOWING it was possible.

Your mindset is going to be what brings you success for the long-term. But you must exercise the principles in this book every day, in some way. Celebrate the small and little things, every single day. This is a key part of the exercise principle. Those intentional inspired actions include being grateful, mindful, and full of wonder.

Thank yourself for taking care of your body each day and making choices that show how much you love yourself. If you ended the day and met your wellness goals, don't blow it off. Get in the mirror and give yourself, a 'you go, girl' or a literal pat on the back. Whatever lets you acknowledge yourself.

Be mindful of the small wins. You went for the apple. You took the stairs. You parked further away in the parking lot. You said no to the extra slice of cheesecake. And be full of wonder about what else is possible and what will you be able to do tomorrow. What are your body and your mind and your spirit capable of? Ask yourself often and with an optimistic energy, 'what else is possible?'

Exercise for Wellness and Fitness

Being active in our daily lives is one of the best medicines for health and longevity. Adding resistance or weight training to your exercise routines is proven to have health benefits that go beyond healthy muscles and bones.

It also adds more protein in the brain which can help protect against later issues such as dementia. Oh, and the benefits to skin. Protein supports the body's production of collagen so if you want more youthful skin, eat your protein. Strength training has been called the fountain of youth because when you nourish your body to increase your strength it gets the nutrients it needs to keep your body humming in other ways.

So yes, you'll be better guarded against falls and bone injuries, but you may also notice other improvements.

Exercise is known to help boost mood and lower depression because we release tryptophan when we work out and our brain uses this amino acid to make serotonin.

Some other benefits of strength training include:

- Improving bone health and prevent osteoporosis

- Reducing symptoms like hot flashes

- Improving sleep quality

- Boosting mood and energy levels

- Maintaining muscle mass and metabolism

In addition, regular exercise, according to the United States Centers for Disease Control and Prevention (CDC) helps prevent or manage many health problems and concerns, including:

- Stroke

- Metabolic syndrome

- High blood pressure

- Type 2 diabetes

- Depression

- Anxiety

- Many types of cancer

- Arthritis

- Falls

It can also help improve cognitive function and helps lower the risk of death from all causes.

As we age, our fitness goals may change. Perhaps being swimsuit sexy isn't a priority, but being able to pick up a new grandchild or keep up with your daily activities is. Sure, I wanted to look nice in a swimsuit, but feeling good and functional in my body is the priority!

Your reasons for being fit and healthy could be as big as wanting to get back into the sports of your younger years, exploring new sports and fitness activities, or being able to go on long walks in nature, or not tire from long days visiting tourist attractions when you're traveling.

How does your fitness allow you to function and thrive in your ideal life?

Getting older is a blessing. We're here to live and experience with more wisdom. However, as some of us may have seen in our own lives, as women there is also ageism and assumptions about what we're capable of doing. We can put to rest the old ideas, my friend.

Gone are the days of having to accept that we're done at middle age or that we're destined to be frail old ladies. That can happen, but we don't have to let it happen.

Women like Ernestine Shepherd, a woman who didn't start bodybuilding until her late fifties. She earned the world record for being the oldest bodybuilder when she was seventy-seven. At the time of this writing she still competes.

Halle Berry, a well-known American actress, born in 1966 has maintained her fitness through regular exercise, including resistance training, and a healthy diet.

Jennifer Lopez, an American actress, singer, and dancer (for those who remember In Living Color) also looks amazing in her fifties through a combination of regular exercise and a thoughtful diet.

You don't have to aim for their level of fitness. It may even be unrealistic for most women, but I wanted to share some examples of what is possible for us and that we don't have to settle for bodies that don't meet our needs. We can improve how we age even if we aren't professional athletes or stars.

With intentional exercise and fitness activities we can combat the deterioration of our body, mind, and prevent ailments that perhaps our mothers and grandmothers didn't have the means or knowledge to prevent. We won't suffer because of not knowing, not if you've got this book.

You saw the list of benefits we can get from training our bodies and functional fitness has the focus of preparing our bodies for daily living into our older age. Being as physically independent as possible for as long as possible is a goal for me. What about you?

Yes, you'll likely lose extra pounds, especially when you pair exercise with the principles of nourishment I share, but you'll also get stronger, improve your cardiovascular health, increase your flexibility, and general mobility. These are things we need to protect our health as we age.

You Can Do This

There are many reasons we don't exercise or stick with a fitness routine. It can feel overwhelming to fit it into our lives.

The time commitment can seem like too much, especially when it takes time to see progress. We might feel that starting means making a long-term commitment to something that we've failed at before. And no one likes to fail. But when it comes to our wellness, we may need to fail sometimes, but we fail forward. We learn through what works and doesn't work.

We've all been on this ride before, but perhaps we didn't strap ourselves in, and the minute it got bumpy we fell off. Strap in, love. It might get bumpy and there may be some twists, turns, and even a few loops. But all that adds to the fun and the adventure.

I want you to have a rich and epic life and that means taking care of yourself and showing up for yourself in ways you may not have done ever, or maybe not in a long time.

Love, you can do this. Even if you've never done it before. Even if you've tried and failed. You can do this. Why? Because your reasons will be bigger and it's about a life of fitness and health and wellness and not about a diet or being deprived.

No one wants to be deprived or stressed out trying to be healthy. That will wreck your gut, set you back, and have you yanking that seatbelt off before this ride even gets its speed up.

Whether you choose to get fit on your own or work with someone, this chapter will help you get started, wherever you are, in as little as twenty minutes.

Walk It Out

You'll notice that walking is coming up again. Another fun fact–my later-in-life novella romantic comedy book series is called The Walking Club because I wanted to include walking. I mentioned in the prior chapter that walking can give us some stress relief, but most of us know it's great for exercise.

It's just that many of us may think of striding along quickly as the way to do it.

As women in our middle and later years, the most powerful thing you can do for your physical fitness is to walk. But we're not talking power-walking. We need to spend most of our walking time moving at a comfortable or even slow pace for longer distances.

Aim for 8,000 to 12,000 steps per day. In a National Institutes of Health study, in JAMA, of more than 4,800 adults over forty years of age, walking 8,000 steps or more daily was associated with a fifty percent decreased risk of death over the next decade, compared to those who walked 4,000 steps or less. When the number of steps went to 12,000 the decrease in risk went up to sixty-five percent. Not bad for walking.

If you haven't been walking, my suggestion is to aim for more steps than you're currently taking and then to work your way up a little each day and each week. I like the 80/20 rule here. Can you reach the step goals eighty percent of the time? If not immediately, can you work up to meeting it eighty percent of the time? That's getting to 8,000 steps eight of every ten days.

If you're sitting at your desk all day you can work in extra steps by getting up every hour to walk somewhere or do anything for a minute or two. You need that break anyway to move your body and keep your hips and joints from getting stiff.

Walking is what our ancestral women did constantly. We were made to walk and we can enjoy the benefits of walking as we age because it's easy on the joints and bones. Add a couple of water bottles or a resistance band and you can enjoy a full body workout, even if it's a lightweight one.

The goal is to enjoy generally easy walks that don't put a lot of stress on your body. If you're already athletic or have been working out, your body can handle more stress than if you're just starting on your wellness journey. We don't want to set back our mojo by doing too much too soon. Remember, progress and consistency.

When you pair walking with the workout below and a healthy diet filled with whole foods, your fitness level will go up and your body's stress levels will go down.

If you can't fit these many steps in every day, aim to reach these step goals on days you don't do a regular workout. You can aim for two to three strength-training workout days and three to five days where you walk.

Remember, every step counts, including those you take in daily life, so try parking in the farther end of the parking lot when you're running errands, walk the dog an extra five minutes, and try taking the stairs when you can.

SIT and Lift

Regular physical activity, particularly weight-bearing exercises like strength training, can help reduce the effects of menopause. That means that if you are yet to hit the menopause window, you can prevent some of the effects in the first place! Studies by the American College of Sports Medicine show it helps maintain bone density, improve cardiovascular health, and boost mood. And a 2019 study published in the journal Menopause found that strength training helped maintain bone density in postmenopausal women.

This is especially important because menopause can lead to a decrease in estrogen, which can speed up bone loss. Strength training helps counteract this by stimulating the bones and muscles, leading to a stronger and healthier physique.

Women are often loath to lift heavy. Our society has gotten used to seeing women age with little grace, demeaning both our silver hairs and strength. But those things can be a beautiful part of this phase of our lives. Let the color of your hair be up to you and let your strength and body serve you.

Physical strength will help you have a better quality of life and keep doing the things that bring you joy, whether it's gardening, traveling, doing sports with friends, or playing with grandchildren.

Not to mention the confidence boost that comes with looking good and feeling strong. We can redefine what it means to age as a woman – strength, power, confidence, and good mojo are all part of what we can have.

BEFORE YOU CONTINUE!

Before starting a new fitness or exercise routine, **please do a personal fitness assessment and talk to your physician** to ensure you're physically ready.

Burn Fat and Build Muscle

Incorporating exercises into your routine that support balance, flexibility, mobility and your cardiovascular health. I include a sample SIT training session as an example and starting point. You can also order one of my ready-made exercise plans or work with a professional trainer. Though it can seem like exercise can be the cure for poor health and fitness, it cannot make up for poor nutritional habits.

One order of medium fries of about four ounces is approximately 365 calories. Someone weighing 180 pounds would need to walk an hour and forty minutes at a moderate pace to burn off just one order of medium fries. And the calories aren't nutrient dense so they don't serve your overall health needs as much. This doesn't mean you can never have fries, just that you may need to be mindful and balanced.

High Intensity Interval Training using Sprint Interval Training

To get the most out of your training, add cardio-vascular training into the mix. I enjoy the version of HIIT that I use that incorporates quick bursts of cardio followed by medium to low intensity resistance moves.

These moves may also incorporate compound movements or be simpler. They are certainly not the only moves you can choose for your exercises. This example includes moves that don't require more than bodyweight, dumbbells, or resistance bands.

You're going to push yourself hard for 30 seconds. Think up to 85% of your maximum heart rate. To calculate your maximum heart rate, subtract your age from 220. If you have a heart condition, diabetes, or cardiovascular health concerns you will need to adjust for this. **Always consult with a physician before beginning an exercise program.**

Once you've done your hard 30 seconds, you'll do an easy to moderate 30 seconds of one of the moves. The idea is not to rush through these but to be intentional about the mind and body connection.

Pick a move that you can do while keeping your form for 20 to 30 seconds. Choose 1 to 2 moves from each 30 second split shown below, per set. Try to switch up for the 2nd set to work different muscles.

Hard 30

- Elliptical

- Run on treadmill

- Run in place

- Jumping Jacks

- Box Jump (use one you can safely jump on and off of 6"-24")

- Run up a hill (pair with walking down the hill)

Easy/Moderate 30

- Dumbbell Bicep Curl

- Dumbbell Bicep Curl to Overhead Press

- Dumbbell Squats to Overhead Press

- Dumbbell Bench Press

- Dumbbell Forward Arm Lift to Side Arm Lift

- Dumbbell Romanian Deadlift OR One Leg Romanian Deadlift

- Walk Down Hill

How to Do the SIT Session
Example Set (Beginner):

Jumping Jacks 30 seconds
Dumbbell Bicep Curl 30 seconds
Jumping Jacks 30 seconds
Dumbbell Bicep Curl 30 seconds
Jumping Jacks 30 seconds
Dumbbell Bicep Curl 30 seconds
Jumping Jacks 30 seconds
Dumbbell Bicep Curl 30 seconds
TOTAL TIME: 4 MINUTES

REST: 4 MINUTES (unless did less than 4 minutes then rest equal to time done.)

TOTAL ROUND: 20 MINUTES FOR 3 SETS OR 12 MINUTES FOR 2 SETS

Repeat the set, working up to 3 sets total.

Example Set (Advanced)

Run in Place 30 seconds

Dumbbell Squats to Overhead Press 30 seconds

Jumping Jacks 30 seconds

Dumbbell One Leg Romanian Deadlift 15 seconds each leg

Box Jumps 30 seconds

Dumbbell Bicep Curl to Overhead Press

Run in Place 30 seconds

Dumbbell Squats to Overhead Press 30 seconds

Jumping Jacks 30 seconds

Dumbbell One Leg Romanian Deadlift 15 seconds each leg

Box Jumps 30 seconds

Dumbbell Bicep Curl to Overhead Press

TOTAL SET TIME: 6 MINUTES REST: 4 MINUTES TOTAL ROUND: 26 MINUTES FOR 3 SETS OR 16 MINUTES FOR 2 SETS

Repeat the set, working up to 3 sets total.

Remember you can do moves other than those in the example. The key is to get your heart pumping hard for 30 seconds followed by a 30 second recovery period and then a full recovery period. If you love burpees, go for it!

Adding In a Focused Heavy Lifting Session

If you choose to do a SIT session without weights, you'll want to do some power moves to train your muscles as well. If you're new to working out and training you may do the beginner type moves that incorporate some weights into the easy/moderate periods.

If adding heavy lifting on top of your SIT session, give yourself a break of between four and six minutes between your SIT session and starting your heavy lifting. You can use this time to set up for heavy lifting (this takes time and energy).

If you've been working out a little longer you may be able to add a 15–20-minute strength training session to your workout for maximum benefits.

This is where you'll add your regular strength and weight lifting routine or you can do the power moves (one or all of them depending on where you are and your goals.)

Power Moves

In the powerlifting world there are three primary disciplines to display strength. They are the squat, the deadlift, and the bench press. All three exercises use multiple major muscle groups and are compound exercises. The key is to lift a heavier load than you normally lift in everyday life. I've chosen moves that you can do at home or the gym using basic equipment like dumbbells. You can also use a barbell.

1. Squats

2. Bench Press

3. Deadlift

First of all, please be careful when executing any of these strength moves. If you have never done them before, work with a trainer or someone who knows what they are doing. Don't bench press or squat without a spotter who can support the weight, especially if you're using a barbell. I was coached by a world-record holding powerlifter to learn how to properly squat, deadlift and bench press.

You can injure yourself if you overload the weights or have improper form. Using dumbbells does decrease the risk but it doesn't make it zero.

After your SIT session you can choose to do all three power moves or perhaps just focus on one each day of training (assuming you do the recommended three days per week of SIT training).

Dividing your power moves up per day might look like this for someone new to training:

- **Monday: Squats** - 2-3 sets of 8 to 15 reps with 2-3 minutes rest between sets

- **Wednesday: Bench Press** - 2-3 sets of 8 to 15 reps with 2-3 minutes rest between sets

- **Friday: Deadlift** - 2-3 sets of 8 to 15 reps with 2-3 minutes rest between sets

After a conditioning period of a month to a month and a half you may be able to add weight and do fewer reps, eventually working up to five reps of five and then four to six sets of three to five reps. This can take time! This will be different if you are already conditioned and experienced.

If you're on a twice per week schedule, rotate through the moves so that you are still getting them all in. You may do squats and bench press this week and then start with the deadlift next week before repeating the rotation, starting with the squat again.

If you've built weights into the SIT session you are still getting weight lifting benefits, it just won't be as heavy, but one heavy lifting move per training day will boost your metabolism and fat-burning capacity. This is part of the secret sauce, love!

How to Choose My Starting Weight?

This will be a bit of trial and error. It's better to go with a medium load and add or decrease it based on how you feel. You should be able to complete the HIIT movements all the way through for nearly all the sets.

For strength training you should be able to complete at least 8 reps of 2 full sets to start. If you find you are struggling with the last couple repetitions on a set, but can still do them and keep your form, stay where you are. Sometimes you have to pause for a few seconds and then continue. If you are straining, don't force it. Don't injure yourself. You can always try a heavier load later.

How Long Should I Do This?

The entire routine for SIT and Heavy Lifting will vary based on how long your sit session is (12 minutes up to 26 minutes) and whether you choose to do one power move or more. At a minimum, your training session will likely be about 30 minutes including:

- 5-minute warm up

- 12-minute SIT

- 4-minute rest

- 5-minute power move session (1 move)

- 5-minute cool down/stretch

This is a total of 31 minutes.

But give yourself a few extra minutes for setting up your SIT area and if you need to warm up or cool down for longer.

If you're signed up for one of my group coaching programs you can also ask for a demo of a movement or exercise. If you ask before the meeting, I can prepare so I can show you live and you can practice. Aside from my Meno Mojo program, my group coaching includes wellness and fitness but that is not the sole focus.

What Happens If I Don't Finish?

Did you do your best to finish the SIT session or heavy lifting session? Do you feel like you exerted yourself more than you usually do? If you feel as if you gave your all to your session without putting yourself at risk of injury, good job.

The idea is not perfect sessions, it's sessions that keep you progressing towards your goal of being fit (and looking and feeling good). If you're doing that and being consistent, congratulations, put down the weights and give yourself a pat on the back.

Make sure you keep track of what you did so that next time you can make progress from there. If you don't track it's hard to see your progress, whether it's two pounds or one additional rep in that first set. I've got a free tracker you can download through BernetteSherman.com/midlif emojo.

Flexibility, Mobility, and Stability

Maintaining our flexibility and mobility during midlife is also important. I mean how much mojo are we going to have if we can't even move? As our hormone levels change, our joints start to stiffen and our muscles lose some of their pliability and flexibility that we had from the estrogen that was once plentiful. It's the same reason our skin is less elastic.

Yep, all of it's connected, but when our muscles and joints are stiff it can impact our daily quality of life.

We can improve our flexibility from the comfort of our home or you can choose to get out of the house, especially for some human interaction. Yoga poses like downward-facing dog and cat-cow, elongate the spine and improve joint range of motion.

You can also hold a standing quad stretch for thirty seconds on each leg to help with tightness in the hips and lower back. I do this and stretch in multiple directions, which helps improve the tightness and my range of motion.

For mobility, focus on dynamic movements that mimic everyday actions. Try toe touches, arm circles, and leg swings to maintain fluidity in your joints. Incorporate ankle circles and knee lifts while standing to improve lower body mobility. My husband laughs, but I'll do moves like this while brushing my teeth. I'll also do body squats and high knees to the front and to the side, and occasionally kickbacks.

The goal is for this period of our lives to be comfortable and for us to stay active. Moving in natural ways as part of our exercise or even micro-fitness moments can help.

When it comes to stability and balance, you can build moves into your everyday activities as well. Again, the time you spend brushing your teeth is ideal for adding in some balance activities. Simply stand on one foot for a few seconds and work your way up to splitting your time balancing on each foot. You can do the same exercise while washing dishes.

If you do the exercise routine above, build balance into the routine by doing dumbbell curls on one leg. You can also do Romanian deadlifts (RDLs) rather than regular deadlifts and shift one leg backwards so most of your weight is on one leg and the other foot is gently on the floor for balance while you do your RDLs.

As you get more balanced, you can lift the toe from the ground so you are balancing on the one primary leg.

Single-leg calf raises with or without a dumb-bell are also a great way to practice your balance. Gently place one hand on a stabilizing surface like a counter to support you. The goal here is not to do this hands-free, but to build your balance and core strength.

When doing stability work your core should be engaged and held firm, while still breathing. Think about pulling your navel towards your spine or bracing yourself for a bundle of energy hug from a favorite small human! You don't necessarily want to clench your buttocks, but you do want to support your entire core, which includes your buttocks.

Having a strong core, flexibility, and mobility will help you continue to enjoy ALL the activities available to you during these freedom years. Even one or two minutes a day will give you results, if you're consistent.

Before moving on to nourishment, I want to add that it's easy to want to push yourself hard. If you're new to exercising or haven't done it in a while, try what I've put above first for a week, then add to it.

Practice rest, reset, and recovery between sessions and if you have a foam roller or a massage gun, use it for muscle soreness and myofascial release. Trust me, it will change your fitness game. Oh, and that foam roller also helps break up cellulite. That tip right there is worth the book! *At least I think so.*

Other Exercise Options

You don't have to do the SIT training sessions. You are always in control and should find ways to move that you enjoy and can be consistent with. If the SIT session is not something you like and trying to time things and stay in that flow is just doing too much, I get it. There are other things you can try. Perhaps you want to dance or make walking your primary form of exercise.

If you choose to walk or dance consider adding ankle or wrist weights. If walking you can also hold hold water bottles. You can even wear a weighted vest to create some weight resistance which is essential.

All of the exercises here are examples over and shouldn't be considered as a training program or plan. To build a balanced body, you'll need to do a variety of exercises over time that target different muscles. Below is another idea for a fifteen to twenty minute workout that only requires dumbbells or resistance bands.

Full-body – Dumbbell Squats and Swings
- Do 1 set of 15 dumbbell squats followed by 1 set of 15 dumbbell swings

- Rest 30 seconds to 90 seconds

- Repeat two times

Upper-body – Bicep Curls to Arnold Shoulder Press
- Use moderate weight dumbbells and do 10 repetitions of bicep curls and transition into an Arnold shoulder press.

- Rest 30 seconds to 90 seconds

- Repeat two times

Lower-body – Leg Extensions with Resistance Bands
- Sit on a chair and wrap resistance band around the bottom of your foot. Hold the other end down with your other foot. Extend your leg in front of you. Do 12 repetitions and then switch legs.

- Rest 30 seconds

- Repeat two times

Whatever you choose to do for exercise and physical fitness is okay. Do whatever literally moves you. My only request is that you add in resistance training to it, and enough to feel it in your muscles. If you aren't feeling it, you are likely not getting enough resistance to get stronger. Other than that, do you!

The Power of One in Exercise

The power of one principle can be applied in a few ways. You can choose to do one thing. You can do one thing for one minute. You can do just one (more) set or rep. The idea is to just start by doing something once. Because if you can do it once, you know you can do it again.

Some examples are choosing to go for a walk once this week. It may be to your mailbox, up the street, or in the park. Perhaps you choose to apply the universal principle of exercise.

What you do isn't as important as that you do it. It could even be to walk in place for one minute. Just choose to do it. Maybe you want to do one sit up. Yes, I literally said one sit up. Or you might try one set of arm curls.

Can you pick one thing you'll tackle that week for one minute, one rep, one set?

The Power of Five in Exercise

Just like the power of one, there is the power of five. When you apply this principle, you're saying a louder yes to yourself. You're saying I am making behavioral changes. If you look at your day and you don't see where you can fit in a half hour to exercise or even a fifteen-minute walk, ask yourself what you can do in five minutes.

Here are some five-minute fitness ideas:

- Walk

- Jog

- Dance

- Do resistance exercises (work different body parts or muscle groups)

- Do jumping jacks or march in place, mixed with core training (planks or bird-dogs or dead bugs)

Midlife Mojo Habit Maker

- What has been your biggest challenge with getting physical activity and exercise on a consistent basis?

- What one thing could you do today to begin adding physical activity or exercise to your life on a regular basis? Can you apply the power of one or or the power of five?

- What one thing can you do in the next week to continue supporting your physical fitness and exercise goals?

- What one thing can you commit to doing, for even one minute, EVERY SINGLE DAY?

Exercise Wrap Up

- What's one thing you learned from this section?

- What one thing stood out the most to you in the Exercise section?

- What one thing do you always want to remember?

Affirmation

I am able to consistently move my body in healthy ways that feel good.

Chapter Six

Nourishment

When people ask me what I did for my diet, I tell them that I was disciplined with what I ate and how much. I paid close attention to my macronutrients and used supplements.

I watched when I ate, how I ate, and gave myself grace to not be perfect, but always try to meet some minimum targets. I also used and continue to use the 80/20 rule. My goal was to follow healthy eating and nutritional principles at least eighty percent of the time, giving me twenty percent to play with.

But it wasn't just this. There was also the other side of getting my mind and spirit right to take care of me and help me get better results.

When I think of how we need to nourish ourselves to both lose weight and get back our mojo, I think of the foods and nutrients we feed our body and what we feed our mind and spirit.

Nourishment as a Universal Principle

In order to create the level of change we seek; we have to nourish ourselves using a top-down approach. I believe in the principle, as above, so below. How you nourish your mind and spirit will flow into how you nourish your body.

Prioritize consuming positive and supportive messages from your environment and surroundings so that this is what feeds your mind and spirit. Surround yourself with people, things, and places that uplift and support you in becoming the person you want to be and having the health and wellness you deserve.

When you are going throughout your day, be aware of things that happen and show up or that you do that you've been desiring. It doesn't matter how big or small and it doesn't have to be around losing the extra weight from changes in our hormones and the impact of cortisol. It can be any area of your life. You just want to practice increasing your awareness.

Then you move into gratitude. If you notice these positive and desirable things in your life you can show gratitude for them. When we aren't even aware of them, we ignore them and the Universe says, 'meh, that wasn't important to her.' We want to tell the Universe, 'YES! More of this. I saw what you did there. Thank you!'

Finally, tap into that energy of excitement and joy about your life. All those little things you've started noticing and being grateful for, be excitedly grateful for them. Do happy dances, make up silly, fun and happy songs. Engage some physical aspect of your body with that excitement to get to the emotion – or energy in motion!

When we nourish our minds and spirits consistently it changes the energy around us, and what comes into our lives as well as how we treat ourselves.

While applying some of my tools for shifting and manifestation I noticed that one night when I made popcorn that I knew I didn't need, but was in my twenty percent space, I didn't eat the whole bag!

Now, you might say that's not a big deal. But you don't understand my relationship with popcorn. I own at least five different popcorn makers, not including regular microwave popcorn. It was the one thing that sent me into an emotional cry-fest when I was pregnant with my son because I'd burnt the last bag of popcorn. So, me not finishing the bag was big for me!

Later lying in bed, I was thinking of things to be grateful for that day and checking in on the different areas of how I managed my rest and reset, exercise, and nourishment and was like, 'wait! I only ate half the bag! Yes!!! I am grateful for my affirmation about being a divine magnet for good health, shifting my energy to not desire more than I needed! Thank you!'

I truly felt great and wanted to celebrate the victory and I did. I even did a little happy dance lying in bed, trying not to disturb my husband, of course. But that half-eaten bag meant something and because I noticed it, I could express gratitude for it, and now the universe knows I appreciate being mindful of nourishing my body and enjoying my food and treats, but not in excess. See how that can work?

Nourishment for Wellness and Fitness

As I moved along my journey to getting back my magic and mojo, I learned more about my gut and the microbiome. I won't get into it here as there are entire books dedicated to this topic, written by experts and doctors.

Resources and what we know constantly change and evolve so instead of putting it in this book of principles that should be timeless. Because of this, I share some resources on my website so they can be updated easily.

We can easily overthink nutrition and sometimes that's the approach that's necessary. If you have chronic health conditions that you're managing you might need to use these principles along with guidelines specific to you from a qualified nutritionist, registered dietitian, or doctor. These individuals practice clinically and, in most states, require licensing.

Nutrition coaches, like me, don't prescribe meal plans or specific diets with exactly what to eat.

Instead we coach behaviors, lifestyle changes, and healthy principles. Some individuals will work with a clinical practitioner for specific meal plans and a nutrition coach to help them be successful in implementing that plan along with making lifestyle changes to support lifelong health and wellness.

When we were younger and our bodies were humming along in our prime reproductive years, we had plenty of available hormones, all in balance. That lets us get away with choices and foods that now love to hang out on our waistlines, sap our energy levels, and effect how we generally feel.

Combine this with the histories a lot of us have of dieting and limiting our calories, and we may even have created issues with our metabolism that need healing. This is possible! I didn't realize how much I was restricting my calories until I started aiming to meet my macronutrient and calorie goals and found myself so full I couldn't finish meals!

What I've learned, and research supports, is that carbohydrates have to be managed differently during the menopausal years. We have to be mindful not just of quantity but also of quality. This is why my popcorn habit has been a personal micro-journey of mine.

Most of us know that certain carbs like white rice, white potatoes, and white breads aren't great for managing our weight but does that mean you have to swear off them forever?

The idea of absolutes doesn't fit with my personal philosophy on diet or nutrition. Some reasons you may exclude foods are religious beliefs, cultural beliefs, social, and environmental philosophies. But just because it isn't *always* good for you might not be a great reason.

You may also have health reasons or allergies making it necessary to avoid certain foods. If it's because of health reasons you may want to work with a medical professional, like someone in integrative medicine.

You can also have tests run to determine if you're officially going through or are in menopause and work with a hormone specialist or get hormone replacement therapy if you're finding that even with the tools and principles I share, you're not getting enough relief. We have the medical field for a reason.

The wonders of modern medicine can support a wellness journey when you use it alongside lifestyle changes. To that point there are also pre-scription medications available that promote fast weight loss by decreasing the appetite.

Currently these are primarily the GLP-1 or Glucagon-like peptide-1 agonists drugs. According to the Cleveland Clinic, "GLP-1 agonists are medications that help lower blood sugar levels and promote weight loss."

Some individuals have even reported that this family of drugs has reduced demand for alcohol and drugs. I haven't tried them but if you are dealing with weight that puts your life at risk, you can always learn to practice a lifestyle that supports better health and getting your mojo back while you get the immediate help you need.

At a minimum, follow some of the core principles around getting enough rest, exercise that includes walking and resistance training, and eating mindfully and a diet that has enough protein and fiber from a diverse assortment of fruits and vegetables.

Macronutrients

Macronutrients are the main building blocks of nutrition. Without them you couldn't build tissue or muscle, your brain couldn't function, and your body wouldn't either.

There are three macronutrients, each with a different purpose.

Protein

From the Greek word protos, which means first, is our most important building block of the body. When we eat protein, it gets broken down into amino acids (essential and non-essential) and eventually gets transported to body tissue and into our bloodstream.

Protein is a powerful macronutrient because it can fill in gaps when other nutrients aren't available.

Because of the importance of these amino acids, our body needs to keep them in constant supply. Otherwise, it will start getting it from our muscle and connective tissues, hormones, and other chemicals. Becoming protein deficient can lead to vital functions shutting down.

Carbohydrates

The word 'carbohydrates' comes from carbon and hydrate or water and they're the primary energy source for our body. They can be simple or complex carbohydrates.

Simple carbohydrates are sugars like glucose, fructose, and sucrose. You can think of them like blood sugar, fruit sugar, and table sugar (real table sugar).

Complex carbohydrates are your starches and fibers, usually from plants and vegetables. They're made up of long chain sugar molecules that take longer to break down. They take longer to break down but provide more consistent energy.

Fats

The word "fat" comes from the Old English word "fæt," meaning "vessel" or "container." This is probably from how fat is stored in our body. Fats are also known as lipids and come in three forms. There are saturated fats, unsaturated fats and trans fats. Trans fats are likely what you've heard you should avoid, and it's true. Trans fats are artificially created through a hydrogenation process.

Despite getting a bad reputation, we need fat. They're good for storing energy, insulation of our body, protection, hormone production, and even vitamin absorption.

However, not all fats are the same and because they're calorie dense, both quality and quantity matter.

My Meal Planning and Macronutrients

In order for me to shed weight I personally ate using a macronutrient split of 40P/30C/30F. This is forty percent protein, thirty percent carbohydrate, and thirty percent fat. We need all three plus an assortment of micronutrients.

As I learned more about my body and worked out with heavy weights, I moved the ratio to be approximately 45P/30C/25F. I tried to keep the protein within one to two percent of forty-five percent and within one to two percent for carbohydrates and fats. I did not start out using the hand measuring method so I was using a kitchen scale, measuring spoons and measuring cups. The hand method is shown to be very close to this (and much easier to do).

In order to change your weight up or down you have to change the balance of energy you consume and use. I mentioned earlier that I could hardly finish my food when I started, because I hadn't been giving my body enough energy and it wasn't used to the increase.

When I began eating protein like I'd been eating starchy carbs, I was full and satisfied. It takes protein longer to digest so it stays with us longer. The same is true for fibrous foods.

I had already been picky about the ingredients being mostly clean, though that can be a challenge in the United States and depending on where you live, access to fresh foods is a problem. Highly processed foods are common and come with extra ingredients that are hard for our bodies to process or confuse our body—like sugar and fat substitutes that aren't actually real food.

Now, I was even more aware but not unrealistic. My goal is to have a real life, not deny myself constantly, or have to always tell myself no. I don't want to live in the energy of no. It's not good for my mojo.

Yes just feels better, doesn't it? But to get to the yes, you may need better options than you've had.

I ate six times per day, a combination of smaller meals and snacks. My calories were generally in the 1200-1450 range but with the mix of macronutrients and how often I ate, I never had a chance to get hungry. You may be saying that seems low, but your number will depend on where you're starting.

I also had to plan. It kept me from making impulse choices that usually weren't as healthy for me. When you want a snack and you don't have a go to snack ready, what will you choose? Hungry for dinner and your food isn't already made or only needs reheating?

You're more likely to grab something quick and easy and justify it by being busy or not having time. But if you plan and prepare your meals you take the guesswork out. I had different levels of preparation.

This means you will want to make a list of foods you enjoy, purchase foods ahead of time, and cook them. Planning with your end goal in mind is key. Purchase enough protein and the assorted fruits and vegetables you need to have a good healthy mix. Buy healthy grains and even fully prepare them.

You can portion out your meals and store them in the refrigerator for meals at home or to take to the office. You'll save yourself a few dollars and the stress of having to figure out how to treat your body well when there aren't as many options available around the office.

Some meals I prepped and put in single serve containers like premade tuna salad with low carb wraps for lunch. Or chicken breast and sweet potatoes and broccoli portioned out into single serve containers. I kept cottage cheese with frozen peaches I could quickly put together when it was snack time. And my last snack of the day was usually yogurt. Sometimes I would add a little protein powder or blueberries based on my full day's macros.

Because I am not a nutritionist or dietician, I can't tell you exactly what to eat. However, I can tell you to be where you are and find foods that are good enough, leave you satisfied, and your body feeling good.

Do You

Let me pause here because this is important. Don't let anyone make you feel bad because your kitchen isn't stocked with one-hundred percent grass fed, organic, non-GMO, all natural, ethically sourced everything. Just don't. Unless they are literally giving you the money to buy your groceries and helping your shop for them, the decisions are yours. I talk about your truth in the Truth chapter but being in your truth when it comes to what you eat, specifically, deserves attention.

One thing to consider when changing behaviors is what is the next best option for you? And I say 'for you' because your next option may be different than mine, your friends, or someone you follow online.

Maybe it's going from no vegetables at dinner to having fried okra instead of fries. Perfect? No, but it is progress and that means you're moving in the right direction.

What nutritional choices are you making on a regular basis that you can make a small tweak to? Instead of a fried chicken sandwich, perhaps the grilled chicken sandwich? Going from canned vegetables to frozen? From frozen to fresh? From fresh to farm-fresh? So many options!

But maybe they're not all available to you and the last thing we want to do during this time of our lives is to give ourselves another reason to feel stressed. So my friend, if grabbing a healthy salad (with protein) at lunch is the only thing you can commit to doing for your diet then do it and be consistent with it. Change nothing else and after a week or two you might notice you feel better.

Most people want to go towards their diet goals at one-hundred miles an hour but they've never run more than fifty miles an hour. It's like being a sprinter and deciding you're jumping into a half-marathon, without training.

You're going to have to prepare yourself in mind, spirit, and body to be successful. And you'll have to be patient while you learn your body in a new way, explore what she's capable of, and push through the setbacks and challenges that will come up.

Nourishment In Action

Please take care of what you're feeding your body. It's your physical fuel for living. This is maybe the most difficult subject to address, because for every person, there's an opinion, a cultural norm, and emotional connections to food.

Even with that, we can have power over what we put into our bodies while still being in alignment with our truth, what we love, and being present in our bodies and our divine feminine energies. We can absolutely be about the 'yes' and the 'and'.

There are so many topics I could cover in this section but I am going to touch on four main things:

- How much to eat

- What to eat

- When to eat

- How to eat

How Much to Eat

In the certification program I went through to become a nutrition coach, we put away the scales and measuring spoons in favor of something most of us always have with us. Our hands. Hand-sized portions are surprisingly accurate when it comes to calories and macronutrients.

In order to manage our macronutrient intake we use our hands to measure servings of proteins, carbohydrates, and fats.

You can find guides online, but here are the basics:

Palm: Approximately 3 ounces of protein.

Fist: About 1 cup of non-starchy vegetables.

Cupped hand: Roughly 1/2 cup of carbohydrates.

Thumb: Equivalent to about 1 tablespoon of fat.

Women wanting to maintain their current weight can generally eat calories at a rate of ten times their weight. So if you weigh 180 pounds you would eat about 1,800 calories per day. BUT, if you're in the menopause window or close to it, these numbers don't always hold true because food affects us differently. Please read the section in this chapter about when to eat.

Even with this caveat, this is a good baseline to start from if you haven't been tracking your food intake. And tracking is important when trying to lose, gain, or maintain your weight. It's estimated that we Americans estimate how much we eat incorrectly by about 1,000 calories– usually on the side of underestimating.

To do a calorie reduction you might start at eight or nine times your weight. So that 180-pound woman would eat approximately 1,440 to 1,620 calories daily. A woman trying to gain weight would use a factor of 12x to start. The same 180-pound woman would be aiming for 2,160 calories daily.

Not everyone burns fat and calories at the same rate. I talk about how you may need to adjust this based on your body type in the Truth chapter.

But these aren't empty calories. We have to be intentional and thoughtful about the quality, quantity, and mix of foods we're using to fuel our bodies.

If you're working out with weights to add more lean muscle, you'll want a slightly different mix than if you're doing light weights and mostly walking. However, most women aren't getting enough fiber or protein, so please pay attention to the targets to aim for in the section below.

What to Eat & Macronutrients

According to the 2012 research by Jakubowicz, macronutrient makeup can impact hunger, satiety, and weight loss maintenance.

In the research she shared that those who ate a low carbohydrate breakfast lost more weight initially but regained the majority back by the sixteen-week follow-up.

The group who ate a high carbohydrate **and** protein breakfast not only maintained weight loss but lost on average more than six additional pounds at follow-up. Here's to life with the **and**!

If you only watch two things, I encourage you to be mindful of your protein intake and your fiber intake. If you started with these two things, you'd see an improvement in how you feel and how you look.

Get Plenty of Protein

Protein has been associated with greater satiety and it digests slower than fat or carbohydrates, keeping us full longer. It's also a key building block for muscle growth, made up of essential and nonessential amino acids we need to build and maintain muscle, for tissue growth and repair tissue, keep your skin and hair looking good, and your brain powered. Without enough protein you will literally (over time) fall apart.

During the menopausal years you'll likely need more protein to keep and build muscle. An easy way to think about how much protein to get is to try to get as many grams of protein as your ideal body weight.

A woman who has an ideal body weight of 150 pounds would consume 150 grams of protein. It is a lot and requires being intentional. If this ratio is too much, try to aim for a minimum of .8 grams per pound of your ideal body weight. In this case the 150-pound woman would aim for 120 grams of protein daily.

It can be more complicated when we start thinking about whether you only want to lose ten pounds and keep muscle, lose ten pounds and gain muscle, or gain weight and add muscle at the same time, or simply lose weight and muscle isn't something you're considering. You'll want to consult with a fitness professional or nutrition coach to figure out what might work best for you.

Pay attention to what types of proteins you eat. Lean proteins are better and they're important for building and repairing tissues, including your muscles. They also support immune function and help with weight management. Also watch when you eat these since timing can impact how well your body uses the protein.

Lean protein is essential for building and repairing tissues, supporting immune function, and aiding in weight management. Here are some excellent options:

- *Poultry*: Chicken breast (skinless) and turkey breast (skinless)

- *Fish and Seafood*: Salmon, tuna, cod, shrimp, halibut, tilapia

- *Beef*: Lean ground beef (90% lean or higher), sirloin steak, and round steak

- *Pork*: Loin and tenderloin

- *Dairy*: Greek yogurt, cottage cheese, and low-fat milk

- *Plant-Based*: Tofu, tempeh, lentils, chickpeas, beans (black, kidney, pinto, etc.), edamame, and seitan

- *Eggs*: Egg whites (these are a staple in my refrigerator!)

Eat Plenty of Fiber, Including Colorful Fruits and Vegetables

I'm sure you've heard it a million times by now in your life, but we really do need to eat our veggies. One reason is because we need our fiber. If you haven't been a fan, aim to add one serving of vegetables (about one fist size) to one or two meals per day, above what you've been doing.

Women need approximately twenty-five to thirty-five grams of fiber daily. Nutrition.org suggests twenty-five grams while Precision Nutrition suggests thirty to thirty-five grams daily. Most of us are only getting half of the lower number, if that. The men in your life need even more!

Already eating those veggies? Great! See if you can eat across a rainbow of colors between Sunday and Saturday. You'll get an even better assortment of nutrients, vitamins, and minerals.

High-fiber, low-glycemic fruits and vegetables help remove bile salts from your intestine, lower cholesterol, improve digestion, and can help control blood sugar levels, amongst other things. Some sources of fibrous vegetables include:

Fruits: Apples, berries (blueberries, raspberries, strawberries, blackberries), citrus fruits (oranges, grapefruit, lemons, limes), pears, plums, and avocado

Vegetables: Broccoli, brussels sprouts, carrots, cauliflower, celery, cucumbers, eggplant, green beans, leafy greens (spinach, kale, lettuce), peppers (bell peppers), and zucchini

One thing to consider is that the glycemic index can be influenced by factors like ripeness and cooking methods. It's generally recommended to focus on consuming a variety of these fruits and vegetables as part of a balanced diet.

Eat Whole Foods When Possible

When you can, reach for foods that are eaten in as close to the form they were created. The more processed foods are, the harder they are on your digestive system and often contain much more added sodium and sugars than needed.

It's important to incorporate nutrition into any wellness program. In fact, I would say that what you put into your body is worth significantly more as a percentage of your wellness lifestyle, than your exercise.

If you're working with a trainer who doesn't provide this coaching, consider seeking out additional support to ensure you have a balanced path to creating the healthy body you need to keep you moving gracefully and with strength to and through your freedom years.

When to Eat

Breakfast is the first intake of calories after our fasting period that happens usually after extended sleep. Most people eat breakfast after waking up in the morning. Shift workers may not, and they deal with the effects of not eating meals in alignment with natural human circadian rhythms. The information I've prepared is meant for people who follow a typical pattern of sleeping at night and waking in the morning.

There are research articles that say that the fast is broken when we intake our first calories. That could be coffee with cream and sugar, a glass of orange juice or tea with milk and sugar. It could be a full-on meal or something in between.

Other research does not count a beverage like coffee or tea when taken without sweeteners or cream or milk. So, if you're one of the six people in the world that drinks black coffee straight - it's not breakfast, and I've got my eye on you.

I should also mention that there is much more research out there on meal timing and nutrient timing in general, under the developing field of chrononutrition. Doing this research had me geeking out a bit but I'll try to keep it simple for you.

Now that we've got that down, let's get on with it.

Breakfast Timing

Since breakfast is the first meal of the day, it reasons that it would be relatively early. But what does early mean?

Kelly et al (2020) conducted a small sample research study of Caucasian adults between fifty-one and sixty-three with four males and two females who were ages fifty-seven and sixty-three. This study included timing of meals. The study showed that breakfast had a positive impact on fat breakdown when taken over a two- and one-half day study period. The participants had the same meals but one group had breakfast and no late-night snack and the other had a late-night snack but no breakfast.

One of the important discussions in the above-mentioned study was the impact of the same meal, taken at different times (breakfast or as a late snack) on fat breakdown (lipid oxidation) while the subjects were sleeping. Those who ate the breakfast meal at breakfast had more fat breakdown.

In a study by which included a review of existing literature along with original research, they conducted a large study of over 200,000 individuals in the United Kingdom. In this study they found that breakfast timing was influenced by heredity in fifty-six percent of individuals. This means that they were predisposed (more inclined) to eating at a certain time or within a certain amount of time of waking.

Although this study wasn't able to show whether breakfast skipping was the cause, it did note that skipping breakfast was linked to obesity. This could be due to the impact skipping breakfast has on total fasting time and how that total fasting time affects our metabolism. *If we extend fasting time, we may make up for it later, in other ways as other studies show.*

On the other hand, eating breakfast too early can also have negative effects because it may interfere with the natural cycle of melatonin. Some people have longer periods where melatonin is high and if breakfast is eaten while melatonin is still high it can increase metabolic risk (Lopez-Minguez et al 2019). You're probably thinking, this is double-talk and not helpful. But bear with me as we will come back to this before I'm done.

Early Birds and Night Owls (The Chronotypes)

It was shown by Lopez-Minguez et al that our chronotype may also affect our breakfast timing. Some of us are morning chronotypes or early birds, functioning and being active earlier in the day. Others are evening chronotypes or night owls, with our best functioning and activity late in the day or at night. These early birds and night owls have different experiences with the effects of meal timing.

The night owl (evening chronotype) who has high caloric intake within two hours of going to bed is five times more likely to be obese. The early bird (morning chronotype) who has a high calorie intake within two hours of waking up is half as likely to be obese (Lopez-Minguez). *Yes, it makes that much of a difference! I told you I would come back to that with a clearer message.*

Eating Breakfast in General

Throughout the research it's generally agreed that eating breakfast yields better outcomes than not eating breakfast () as far as how the body responds to later meals, the glucose and insulin levels after the breakfast timeframe, and in body mass indices (BMI).

While BMI is arguably not the best measure it is one that has been used in research for decades and therefore can be compared. This may differ by chronotype but, generally, those who eat breakfast have a lower chance of being overweight or having obesity.

In a study with ninety-three women averaging within seven years of forty-six, found that those who ate a high calorie breakfast compared to high calorie dinner had more weight loss compared to the women who ate a high calorie dinner. According to Jakubowicz 'fasting glucose, insulin, and ghrelin were reduced in both groups.

However for the group with a high calorie breakfast there was a *significant* decrease on all of these measures plus on HOMA-IR a measure of how well their bodies responded to . In this research study by Jakubowicz women ate breakfast at 8am.

In a later study found that diabetic individuals who skipped breakfast had a higher rate of postprandial (post-eating) hyperglycemia (high blood sugar) (PPHG) despite having the same carbohydrate makeup in their dusk meal as those who had it in the morning. Having the higher calorie breakfast had a benefit on "weight loss, appetite, and reduction of PPHG".

The findings again suggest breakfast can support a heavier calorie and carbohydrate load compared to later meals. So if you're going to lean towards a bigger carb-loaded meal, breakfast works better for it than a late meal.

In an observational study by made up of individuals over forty and who were predominantly women (71%), they found that the twenty-two individuals who skipped breakfast had "significantly higher levels, higher body mass indices (BMI), and later MSF (mid-sleep time on free days)". The Reukrakul study also associated skipping breakfast with the night owl chronotype.

A review of other research findings with predominantly female populations of diverse ages shows that eating breakfast has a positive benefit to insulin levels, satiety, BMI levels and weight loss from eating a higher calorie breakfast. This is compared to skipping breakfast or eating the higher calorie meal late in the day or at night within two hours before bed.

Other discussions of chronotypes break people into more than these two groups and label us by other animals, but for the purpose of the information I'm sharing, the two primary types should be enough.

Generally proteins take about two to six hours to digest, depending on how complex the source is. Eating protein throughout the day can aid in protein synthesis, starting with breakfast. A breakfast with healthy lean proteins and nutrient dense carbohydrates has the best potential for keeping you satisfied until the next meal and the healthier carbs can impact post-eating blood sugar levels as well. Generally women who want to maintain or build muscle (which is ideally all of us) need at least .8 grams of protein per pound of our ideal body weight. If you can get 1 gram per pound, even better.

Research shows that our bodies tend to do well with eating proteins during the day, carbohydrates earlier in the day, and fattier foods later in the day. With this we do best to avoid heavy meals and high calorie meals late in the evening (). This is contrary to our culture in the United States and in many parts of the world where either a late lunch or dinner are the main meal.

They also found and reconfirmed that skipping breakfast doesn't necessarily result in weight loss as people will overcompensate for the missed calories later and will do less physical activity throughout the day. Depending on your routines and preferences, making either breakfast or lunch, at a reasonable time, your main meal may help with glucose and insulin levels along with weight management.

Personally, I have recently tested having more carbs early in the day and easing off later in the day. Particularly with popcorn. Previously I would make a nice huge bowl of popcorn in the evening and feel bloated in the night and morning. It was great going down but didn't land very well.

I shifted my popcorn party to before two o'clock in the afternoon and paired it with a lean protein source or sardines (I admit I love them and they are an underrated superfood). I have the occasional later evening popcorn, as I mentioned earlier, but try not to make that the habit.

I would literally gain a pound overnight with my evening popcorn snacks and feel bad in my body. By adjusting the time, I have eliminated the morning bloat and bad feeling and my body processes the carbohydrates and fiber in the hours I'm still awake.

The other thing I do with my carb-heavy days is pair them with my HIIT/SIT workout days which amps my metabolism up for several hours-the hours I'm doing my happy snacking.

Now back to what you came for.

Putting it Altogether

So do you think you can skip breakfast and get positive benefits? Unfortunately, nah sis. It can seriously backfire. Kinda like diet sodas and fat-free foods with substitutions to make you think you're getting the real stuff. You can't fake it until you make it with your body and in midlife is when everything starts catching up with us.

Don't get overwhelmed, because you can start with one thing. Breakfast.

Breakfast is the start of your day and can set a positive tone for your body and your circadian rhythm for the rest of the day, keeping your hunger levels, insulin, and glucose levels in check and providing enough energy for you to be more physically active during the day.

Yes, breakfast is a key part of a self-care routine for each twenty-four-hour cycle. I guess mom was right again. Breakfast is the most important meal of the day

Here are a few research-supported takeaways and tips for eating and timing of breakfast.

- Eating a higher calorie breakfast compared to saving your biggest meal for dinner can help in weight loss and weight management.

- Eating most of your carbohydrates earlier compared to at dinner or during late night snacks is shown to help with insulin, glucose, and weight.

- Eating protein along with carbohydrates for breakfast can provide better satisfaction and keep you fuller longer.

- It is recommended to eat within two hours of waking.

- It is best to avoid eating a high calorie meal within two hours of going to sleep.

- A proper night's sleep helps the body manage and process the nutrients, reset internal clocks and the circadian rhythm, and prepare for the next twenty-four-hour cycle.

- Those who eat based on being night owls have a higher risk of being overweight and having obesity compared to those who eat based on being early birds.

It's not too late to start making healthy lifestyle adjustments. I made a big change at forty-seven and I am still tweaking and finding what works for my changing body during the time leading up to my freedom years.

In addition to what the science says, listen to your body and its cues. Feel for hunger cues versus cues that masquerade as hunger such as boredom, anxiety, nervousness, depression, stress, etcetera.

If you are unaccustomed to eating breakfast, start small and test out different timing windows. Planning consistent meal times trains your body to process food and helps regulate your internal clock. Randomly eating actually can cause internal confusion, improper food storage (or simply putting some of your food calories into storage when you'd rather they be broken down and used), and slowing of your metabolism.

Another easy thing to do, besides eating breakfast, is to start paying attention to what you're already doing. You can try keeping a food journal for a full week and include how you feel before and after meals, being very mindful of your SHMEC (stress, hunger, mood, energy, and cravings) each day and throughout the day. You can grab a free food log at BernetteSherman.com/midlifemojo.

This will give you lots of information specific to you and your body and allow you to adjust as needed. But this isn't necessary to get started and you can always do this later if you want.

The bottom line is to eat a balanced and nutritious breakfast within a couple of hours of waking in order to send good fuel and food signals to your body for the rest of the day.

How to Eat

How we eat can have an impact on how much we wind up eating and what we wind up eating. This topic could be a small book on its own and

I've already given you a small book on nourishing your body, but how to eat for better nourishment and satisfaction deserves some space.

Since this isn't a nutrition guide, I'll give you another great tip to help with your nutritional goals. It's to be mindful of what you're eating, where you're eating, and even how you're eating.

Here are three simple yet interrelated habits that you can start applying immediately to how you eat meals.

1. *Eat slower.* There are rich flavors, textures, aromas - all to scintillate us. Chew your food well and put your fork or spoon down between bites. Try to pace yourself with the slowest eater at the table. It can help to eat at a table and when possible, eat as a social experience and engage in conversation.

2. *Eat until you are eighty-percent full or comfortably satisfied.* Don't eat until you're full. Your brain doesn't get the message that your belly is full until about twenty minutes later. Don't immediately go back for seconds or thirds. Let your food digest some and listen

to your body to feel if more food is needed or if you're satisfied.

3. *Eat mindfully and with few distractions.* When we slow down, it allows for a better connection between our mind and body. Eating should be a sensory experience and smelling, tasting, and feeling your food in your mouth should be part of it. Don't rush the sensations by taking large bites.

Cheat Days

There's no need for a cheat day when you realize that good, tasty foods and enjoying meals is part of a full life experience. I don't do cheat days but I do flex days or flex meals.

Before blowing five days of progress in one meal or an entire day (or weekend), remember your goals, and the basic principle of doing little things to make progress. Perhaps rather than eating everything you didn't have this past week; you pick a couple of things to indulge in and be flexible about when you do it. One meal? Over one day? Over one weekend?

Progress is day by day but we need flexibility to live real lives and accountability to our goals at the same time. If that second piece of cheesecake is calling tonight, how will you flex your nutritional goals tomorrow?

Remember, there's a certain amount of "money" in the bank and you may spend more today than yesterday but when you spend more than you have, you get overdrawn. And those fees add up and are painful.

You've got goals and you deserve to reach them.

The Power of One in Nourishment

The power of one principle in nourishment still has several ways you can apply it. You can be very creative. For example, maybe it's adding one vegetable or fruit to one meal. Or choosing one day a week to avoid fried foods. Eating one bite at a time, thoroughly chewing, savoring, and swallowing before taking the next bite (you might be surprised if you try this one).

The power of one principle might even be, waiting one minute and doing something else before going back for seconds or immediately refilling a sugary beverage. It gives us a chance to slow down or try something new.

The Power of Five in Nourishment

Using the power of five in nourishment can really help us slow down and be more mindful. I like to use the power of five when I might be in the mood to eat my feelings, or bury my stress in comfort foods. I know I'm not the only one who's wanted to eat a bunch of starchy carbs, sweets, and fatty foods that just make us feel good in the moment, but then sap away more of our mojo.

By using the power of five here you can slow down and really let yourself connect with your body. You can do a body scan, journal about your day and what happened that day, and how you're feeling, and even take a check of your SHMEC. You may find clues about why you suddenly have that craving for butter pecan ice cream and a big bowl of popcorn. I may be projecting, but I'm not wrong.

You can also use the power of five in nourishment to count that you've included a variety of at least five different fruits or vegetables in your day or that you had five full servings of fruits and vegetables. Perhaps you want to use the power of five to eat more slowly and mindfully.

If you're a faster eater, force yourself to slow down so that you are sitting down and eating five minutes longer. If it usually takes you fifteen minutes to eat dinner, eat slowly enough to stretch it to twenty. Or you might decide to wait five minutes before getting dessert or filling your plate with seconds. The added benefit is that it takes about twenty minutes for our brains to tell our bellies that we've had enough.

Midlife Mojo Habit Maker

- What has been your biggest challenge with eating a balanced and truly nourishing diet consistently?

- What one thing could you do today to begin eating healthier on a regular basis? Can you apply the power of one or five?

- What one thing can you do in the next week

to continue improving your nourishment, nutrition and dietary habits?

Nourishment Wrap Up

- What's one thing you learned from this section?

- What one thing stood out the most to you in the Nourish section?

- What one thing do you always want to remember?

Affirmation

I nourish my body with healthy, enjoyable foods that support my body and my life.

Chapter Seven

Truth

This is the final principle when it comes to watching your RENT. The truth principle is about acknowledging your individuality, unique needs and desires, and where you are when it comes to wellness and your well-being.

We are all different people with different goals, abilities, and bodies.

What one person does successfully may not apply to you, and vice versa.

As you apply the principles of rest, exercise, and nourishment it should always be through the lens of your truth.

What is real and right for you?

What resonates with your current and desired experience?

How are you doing across all areas of your life? Physical health isn't in a vacuum.

Only you can answer that.

The best way to answer this and to be attuned to your truth is to learn to listen to your body and your intuition. It also requires being honest with yourself and open to seeing the reality of your current situation.

Truth as a Universal Principle

When we think about our curves and all the angles we have, the way we flow, and move in and out of alignment with our truth, we can see how it's not straightforward.

My curves physically, mentally, and spiritually are going to be different than yours. The things that have shifted in my life (and my body) during these middle years may have some similarities to yours.

We're each special and our curves, whether we love them or not, are part of what make us special. Whether we're trying to smooth them out, put them back in place, or amplify them these curves are part of our story.

Like a shero, every curve has a story and so does every curveball! They have literally shaped us into the women we show up as today. Do we have to take all of them with us forward? Absolutely not. But we can take the lessons, the blessings, and whatever else good we can from them as we put our lives and bodies into the shape we want them to be.

Truth can be a tricky concept when it comes to universal principles and how we apply them. Whatever we believe to be true or untrue for ourselves will be OUR truth, but not necessarily THE truth.

Our personal beliefs and the extent to which we believe, think, and act on those beliefs will impact the reality we create. This is why everything that came before this last principle is essential.

If you believe you can lose ten pounds in twenty-eight days that will be your truth. If you don't believe you can do it, that will be your truth.

I believed I could lose eight to ten pounds in a month and thirty pounds in fourteen weeks. I shed thirty-two pounds in twelve weeks.

When you apply these universal principles consistently and show up physically to apply the practical principles, you can be successful in achieving whatever goals you've set for yourself.

Your truth is going to be personal and subjective because no one else is living in your body or inside your head. You get to control the stories you tell yourself and the one you are writing now. You can even learn to rewrite the stories of your life.

With that in mind, ask yourself, what is possible for your health, fitness, overall wellness, and your life?

Do you believe you can have a lifestyle that supports your wellness as you age?

Do you believe you can lose the extra belly fat? Get stronger? Get leaner?

What about having more endurance? Keeping up with your pickleball games? Going for long walks without having to stop every one-hundred yards?

Do you believe you can look great in that dress that's been sitting in the back of your closet for eight years?

What's your midlife mojo, high-vibing, 'I'm that girl' truth?

Truth for Wellness and Fitness

Your Body

All of our curves are as unique as we are. And this is especially true with our bodies. We all look different and that's a beautiful thing about our world. There is diversity in nature and so there is diversity in humans and our bodies. The fact that we aren't all built the same deserves some attention. It's part of your truth, Love.

I'm not going to get into whether you're an hour-glass shape or not, but the ones that apply more to fitness. These are the endomorph, ectomorph, and mesomorph body types.

Endomorphs usually have a rounded body shape with a higher percentage of body fat. They often have wider hips and shoulders and tend to gain weight easily. This body type can often have a slower metabolism which means it's easier for them to store their excess calories as fat.

Ectomorphs will generally be lean and slender which narrow shoulders and hips. Some might describe an ectomorph as having a delicate frame. They actually have a more difficult time gaining weight, even when they eat more calories.

Ectomorphs have a higher metabolism and burn their calories faster. Keira Knightly and Taylor Swift would be examples of ectomorphs. Jennifer Hudson and Melissa McCarthy are examples of ectomorphs.

Mesomorphs are considered the "athletic" body type. They have a well-defined muscular physique with a balanced proportion of body fat and muscle mass. Mesomorphs tend to gain muscle easily and have a moderate metabolism.

Mesomorphs often excel in athletic activities due to their natural physical attributes. However, a mesomorph can get out of balance as well and may not appear as a mesomorph if they've either increased or decreased the balance between exercise and calories taken in. A celebrity mesomorph would be Scarlett Johansson.

How can you tell which body type you are? Trying to figure this out can be tricky and most people won't fall firmly into one type. Just like most other things in life, there is a continuum. At one end you have the super slim model-types who are long and lanky and on the other end you have the rugby player you don't want to match up against.

All are perfectly fine body types. They're just different and must be treated differently. Depending on where you fall, you may have to adjust how you exercise and nourish your body.

Here are a few questions you can ask yourself to get clues about which type you might be.

Bone structure: Are you generally broad-shouldered and wide-hipped (mesomorph), narrow-shouldered and narrow-hipped (ectomorph), or rounder with a wider waist (endomorph)?

Weight gain and loss: Do you easily gain weight and find it difficult to lose (endomorph), struggle to gain weight (ectomorph), or gain and lose weight relatively easily (mesomorph)?

Muscle development: Do you tend to build muscle easily (mesomorph)?

If you're an endomorph you may find that you can't do ten times your body weight to maintain and that nine or nine- and one-half times your body weight is needed and that rather than the minimum 8,000 steps you may need a few more. The ectomorph's experience could be the other way, needing more calories each day and fewer steps and exercise in order to maintain a healthy weight and body composition.

Being fit will look different for each body type. You can be healthy and strong and still not look like the typical fit example. I personally am closer to the mesomorph body type. My husband is closer to the ectomorph with some mesomorph, and my daughter is more of an endomorph.

We can all be healthy and strong while honoring our different body types and needs. I can't eat what my husband eats. Here's a hint—most women can't. Men simply need more calories every day to maintain their body weight and muscle. A recent study showed they actually have to do more cardio to get the same health benefits women get for less. So, there's a plus for us!

When it comes to shapes within these body types there are also differences, but I don't want to get into all the different body shapes there are. I do include information on my resources. There is one important thing I do want to talk about because it can impact our health and for my body shape, it is a risk factor.

Where you carry your body fat can impact your risk for cardiovascular diseases. If you're like me and extra pounds like to find your way to your middle, which is very common in midlife, it can impact our health. This type of fat is stored deep within the abdomen, surrounding organs like the liver and intestines.

Unlike subcutaneous fat (the kind you can pinch), visceral fat is more metabolically active and releases substances that can contribute to heart disease, type 2 diabetes, stroke, sleep apnea, and even some cancers.

One way to see if you're at risk is to get a measure of your visceral fat as well as a waist to hip ratio measurement. You may need a special digital scale for measuring visceral fat, but a tape measure is all you need for the waist to hip ratio.

The bottom line is that you'll need to be honest with yourself while honoring the body you're in. If you're at greater risk of carrying more body fat due to your body type or body shape, that means you'll need to be more mindful of your choices. That doesn't mean anyone can eat with reckless abandon or adopt a lifestyle of inactivity with their main exercise being lifting the remote.

Your body is here to serve you and it's only fair that you return the favor.

Wellness

When we consider wellness, there are many different understandings and the goal of this book is not to define what wellness means or the difference between fitness, wellness, and well-being, but I want to share, briefly, how I look at them and why.

Fitness is the state of wellness within your body, so your physical wellness as a result of your nutrition, physical activity, rest and recovery, and stress management.

Wellness is often thought of as something people do or are actively engaged in, such as having a lifestyle of wellness. Wellness is usually thought of as having many dimensions.

Depending on where you look you may see six dimensions, eight dimensions, ten, or even twelve dimensions of wellness. I like to look at six or eight dimensions of wellness, depending on my reasons. Below I'll discuss eight of them.

You are entering a wellness journey, for example, with a goal of improving your physical health and while you're at it, you'll likely improve your emotional wellness as well.

However, like fitness is an aspect of wellness, wellness is an aspect of well-being.

Eight Dimensions of Wellness

Generally the eight dimensions of wellness are:

Physical

Based on living a healthy lifestyle so you can have a long, full, and happy life while preventing disease and slowing the process of aging through healthy habits. It includes physical activity, healthy nutrition, sleep and rest habits (sleep hygiene).

Emotional

Based on a sense of well-being, including emotional health and mental health, and our ability to be resilient and cope with life stressors and difficulties.

It includes mood, stress management, anxiety, and self-care.

Social

Based on our relationships and interactions with others for socializing, community, and support. It includes speaking with friends and family, being involved in activities with others, and having people we can trust and rely on and who trust and rely on us.

Spiritual

Based on our sense of purpose and meaning and can include our values, beliefs, principles, morals, and ethics. It also includes meditation and prayer, gratitude, self-love and acceptance, mindfulness and peace of mind, spending time in nature, contemplative study, and compassion for ourselves and others.

Intellectual

Based on our creative abilities, intelligence, and expansion of knowledge, skills, talents, and abilities. Intellectual wellness is also connected with our will.

It includes personal and professional development, personal hobbies, community involvement and voluntarism, cultural involvement, and intellectual curiosity.

Occupational (and Vocational)

Based on using our knowledge, skills, talents, and abilities to create a purposeful life and is closely connected to intellectual wellness. This is a case in which intellectual wellness shows up in our lives. It includes work (inside or outside the home), voluntarism, philanthropy, and studying and learning for our occupation.

Financial

Based on being able to fully meet your financial obligations while also being able to enjoy life both in the present and in the future, while feeling secure. It includes understanding money or financial management, being able to budget for living, expenses, and savings, keeping track of earnings and expenses, and having knowledge, skills, abilities to earn money (*I love this one – manifesting money is part of my mojo!*).

Environmental

Based on creating a supportive environment that contributes to your overall wellness and gives you a sense of safety, peace, and wellness. It includes having supportive people around you, having access to and keeping healthy foods, being able to get fresh air, and an environment both in and outside your home to rest and relax. It also includes being able to keep safe from environmental hazards and pollutants.

★★★

You can do a free dimensions of wellness assessment online. There are plenty of them available. I include a link in the resources on my website available at BernetteSherman.com/midlifemojo.

As you can see it covers many of the areas traditionally considered wellness. There isn't a single definition to clearly say the difference between wellness and wellbeing and at this point you'll likely hear them interchangeably. For the scope of this book we're primarily dealing with your physical wellness.

But I realize our physical wellness and what we do to care for it will have a positive impact on other wellness dimensions, especially our emotional wellness and possibly our spiritual wellness. We may even be motivated to improve dimensions of social wellness, intellectual wellness, and occupational wellness when we have newfound confidence.

According to Seong-Hee Ko and Hyun-Sook Kim of Seoul, Korea in their article in Nutrients (2020), *"ovarian estrogens increase the storage of peripheral fat mainly in the gluteal and femoral subcutaneous regions, while androgens—primarily bioavailable testosterones—augment the accumulation of visceral abdominal fat. The marked decrease in estrogen concentrations accompanying relative hyperandrogenism is regarded as the main factor that causes weight gain and redistribution of body fat in postmenopausal women."*

This means that the combination of fluctuating estrogen levels (particular estradiol, E2) combined with the little brother, testosterone, causes more visceral fat in our bellies (the deep fat). The more active little brother, now playing with less present big sisters, is a bit hyper and this combination causes weight gain, especially in our belly area.

Their paper also references a longitudinal community-based Study of Women's Health Across the Nation (SWAN). This study showed that increased combination of the testosterone to E2 ratio is a predictor to obesity and dysregulated lipid metabolism during the perimenopause and menopause period.

When you're listening and tuning into your body there are a few things to keep an eye on. They can give you vital information about your current state and will impact what behaviors you do around rest, exercise, and nutrition.

Check Your SHMEC

SHMEC stands for stress, hunger, mood, energy, and cravings.

Throughout the day you can do a quick SHMEC check. Simply listen to your body and mind about your current level of stress, hunger, your mood, your energy, and the cravings you have.

As you start out you may want to keep a journal and check it when you wake up, sometime in the middle of your day and in the evening. You can do this to get sense for how your SHMEC areas relate to each other.

For example, when you rate your stress at a ten are your cravings also at a ten? When your hunger is seven is your mood at a three and energy at a four? Everything is connected and when you can notice it in your body and make note of it, you'll become more mindful of each of these measures.

Try using a scale of one to ten with one being extremely low and ten being extremely high.

If you find you are consistently ranking yourself low on anything, it's time to dig deeper to figure out what's going on. Are you taking on more stress than you can manage? Are you not getting enough sleep? Under nourishing your body? Overfeeding your body? Overexercising? Not moving enough?

Paying attention to our bodies and their needs are a core part to getting back our mojo and it applies to everything else in our lives. Practice some of the techniques I shared in the mindfulness chapter to tune into your body and the experience your body is having with rest, exercise, and nutrition–both now and when you make changes to support your mojo for life.

Not everything will work for you and there are things you'll discover on your journey that aren't in this book but that will work for you. When our SHMEC isn't in check, we aren't going to show up with our power and magic, ready to live the lives we know are possible.

I mean, that's what you're here for – the mojo.

Watching your RENT helps with getting that mojo back and creating a life where you have the energy and vitality to do the things you said you wanted to do. Remember the goals you had? Remember the vision you have for this phase of life? It is all possible.

The Power of One in Truth

The power of one principle in truth can have many forms. A one-minute check-in with yourself to make sure what you're doing or choosing is in alignment with you and your body's needs is a great example. So is, a one-minute SHMEC check a couple times daily.

The Power of Five in Truth

Using the power of five in truth, like with nutrition, can let us really slow down and be mindful with how we feel, how our body feels, what we need and what our body needs.

A longer body scan, meditation, or deep breathing for five minutes can not only calm our nervous system, but it can help us become aware of what is happening in our lives that may be impacting our mood and stress levels. This is a great time to do a scan of how you feel when you think about each of the main dimensions of wellness.

Midlife Mojo Habit Maker

- What has been your biggest challenge with being in alignment with your truth?

- What one thing could you do today to begin connecting with yourself and your inner guidance on a regular basis? Can you apply the power of one or five?

- What one thing can you do in the next week to continue improving your intuition, self-awareness, or SHMEC?

Truth Wrap Up

- What's one thing you learned from this section?

- What one thing stood out the most to you in the Truth section?

- What one thing do you always want to remember?

Affirmation

I am honest with myself about my body, mind, and spirit including what is true for me, what feels good, what doesn't, and what is in alignment with my goals.

Chapter Eight

What's Next

Your curves are beautiful, my friend. Inside and out and like I said in the Truth chapter, they have helped shape you.

Hold onto what's most beautiful about them and the good things that came with them, even as you re-shape yourself into the next evolution of who you're meant to be in this world. Your divine purpose is calling and it wants the best possible version you can manifest of yourself to show up.

Our physical wellness, and what we do to care for it, will have a positive impact on our other wellness dimensions, especially our emotional wellness and possibly our spiritual wellness. If you want that mojo that gets you up and going to create a life you love during menopause, your body has to work for you.

When you feel good in your body and have that newfound confidence you may even be motivated to improve dimensions of social wellness, intellectual wellness, and occupational wellness.

Some of you may read or listen to this book and skip the questions and exercises, saying that you'll get back to them later. If that's the case, don't get a case of the 'guilts'. How's that going to serve you or keep you from stressing? Go back and do it. It's that simple. No excuses or explanations needed. There's always a day one.

Remember to grab the free four week workbook with the questions I include at the end of the RENT chapters in the bonus materials available at Bernett eSherman.com/midlifemojo. I really encourage you not to skip this part. It'll help you be ready to move forward into what's next for you.

Who Moved My Curves? is more than a book. It's a way you can approach this phase of your life. Like any other rent, we have to pay the RENT of the principles of Rest-Reset, Exercise, Nourishment, and Truth regularly in order to keep whatever we've got. We can't assume we'll do it once and be done. Forgiveness and clearing work have to be a regular part of your routine, just like exercise, and nourishment.

My journey is ongoing too. I don't get everything right all of the time, and I'm fine with that. I don't want to live a life stressing over whether it's perfect. No. I want to enjoy myself while following the basic principles I've laid out for you. They work when you work with them.

Some days I make a big batch of popcorn because my mood is craving comfort. While I might slip into this feeling eating mode for a day, I know I can't stay there. I have also set my weight target, which happens to be slightly higher than my ideal body weight. Why? Because I don't want to live in a state of denying myself. Those couple of pounds are my happy pounds. Think about what that might mean for you.

You can be fit for life and manifest the epic life you love. That's what I sincerely believe.

If you're ready to truly get back your mojo, starting in your body, please follow the guidance in this book and consider getting support.

Remember, you are a divine feminine being and you're worth it.

When we invest in our health and wellness now, we minimize what we have to invest in illness later.

I do offer coaching for women in general who are ready to step into their own epic adventures and rewrite their stories. My next book on healing and mindset will be out in early 2025 and you'll be able to find information at BernetteSherman.com.

In fact starting at BernetteSherman.com will let you access my coaching in general and everything else I offer. You'll also find the resources I mentioned in this book there at BernetteSherman.com/midlife mojo.

My wish for you is to experience a life with more wellness, joy, love, and abundance from this day forward and to never question if you are worthy. Instead it's to wake up every day knowing you deserve to give yourself love, attention, and care so that you can pour into the world from the overflow.

There is so much you have to offer when you can show up confidently, powerfully, and with all of your mojo. Imagine what your life will be like when you embrace this next phase and start your journey to creating your own magic and mojo. There are adventures awaiting. Your divine purpose is waiting too.

You may also be wondering what else you can create and manifest using some of these RENT principles. Let me tell you, love, your body is just the beginning!

I've manifested loving relationships with my children and husband and wealth that will follow my children for generations. As a healer and with self-healing, I've learned to clear old energy and stories, which is an ongoing process. Using what began as the practices I included in my original Creating Miracles program in 2017 I have continued to refine and develop my manifestation practice to the point it is today. You can heal, shift your mindset, and manifest too.

I invite you to join me on your epic journey by joining my EPIC Living group on Facebook. You can find out about programs I have that incorporate these principles and find the bonus resources for getting your mojo back at BernetteSherman.com/

midlifemojo. Your one-page jumpstart guide is on the next page.

You've got things to do, a body to get back, and a life to live.

Now go out there and get back your mojo.

Oh, and while you're at it, share some of that good mojo you're making by rating and reviewing this book on Amazon or wherever you buy books online.

Four-Week Jumpstart Guide

Week 1

- Read through the book and download the bonus materials OR get a journal to write in.

- Do your general measurements of weight and waist to hip ratio measurements.

- Take photos of yourself in fitted exercise clothing – front and side

- Try out each of the mindfulness techniques in chapter four of breathing, body scanning, and walking to aid in stress relief.

- Do the forgiveness and clearing exercise in chapter four.

- Write your exercise schedule down and put in your calendar-block time for it. Make arrangements to secure this time, if necessary.

- Walk or do the SIT session at least once this week. Aim for two physical activity sessions this week.

- Be sure to do post-workout recovery as well such as stretching, hydrotherapy, or foam rolling.

- Determine what you want to eat and how much. Make a shopping list that includes an assortment of healthy foods. Buy groceries and pre-make a few meals you can store.

- Track your food for a week, using the 7-day food journal (in the bonus resources)

- Do a SHMEC check-in daily.

- Give yourself a reward for reading the book and doing the work that supports you and your goals.

Week 2

- Revisit your midlife mojo vision and goals and remember why you're doing this.

- Ask yourself how you like to move.

- What's your general body type? Ectomorph, endomorph, mesomorph? What might this mean for how you move and feed yourself?

- Follow the schedule you created for yourself. How will you remain accountable to show up for yourself?

- Remember to do recovery exercises.

- If you haven't done the midlife mojo habit maker exercises in the Exercise chapter, do them this week.

- Make any adjustments you need to make to your exercise schedule for the upcoming week.

- Review your food journal. What did you find? What needs adjusting?

- On day 14, repeat your measurements and photos.

- Do a SHMEC check-in daily.

- Give yourself a reward for reading the book and doing the work that supports you and your goals.

Week 3

- Follow your exercise schedule and continue to prioritize your self-care (you deserve it!)

- Remember to do recovery exercises.

- If you haven't done the midlife mojo habit maker exercises in the Nourishment chapter, do them this week.

- Plan your meals for the week and do any necessary grocery shopping so you can prepare your meals.

- How can you apply the power of one and the power of five this way in a new way?

- Can you add one more rep, one more set, one more day of exercise?

- Can you add one more vegetable, one more color of vegetable, or more fiber/

- Can you eat slower by five minutes or give

yourself a five-minute body scan before eating at a time that isn't a regular meal time?

- Time for truth.

- What is working well for you? What are your wins, big or small?

- What are your challenges?

- How are you continuing to pay your RENT?

- Do a SHMEC check-in daily.

  - What have you noticed about your body, your mood, your mind, and how you feel?

  - Write all of the answers and thoughts in your journal or workbook.

- Give yourself a reward for reading the book and doing the work that supports you and your goals.

Week 4

- Continue to build habits for rest and reset, exercise, nourishment, and your truth.

  ○ Revisit the midlife mojo habit maker sections for rest-reset, exercise and nourishment for ideas.

- If you haven't done the midlife mojo habit maker exercises in the Truth chapter, do them this week.

- Revisit your vision and goals. Do you want to make changes as you move forward? Go for it.

- Follow your exercise schedule and write in your journal about how you're feeling. The initial discomfort should have eased up by now as you get into a rhythm.

- Plan your meals for the week and do any necessary grocery shopping so you can prepare your meals.

- On day 28, repeat your measurements and photos.

- It's time to celebrate 28 days of getting your body and mojo back. I know it's not easy but you are here and that means you can keep going!

Notes

Rest–Reset Notes

BERNETTE SHERMAN

Exercise Notes

BERNETTE SHERMAN

Nourishment Notes

BERNETTE SHERMAN

Truth Notes

BERNETTE SHERMAN

General Notes

BERNETTE SHERMAN

About the Author

Bernette Sherman is a multi-passionate creative intuitive who uses her gifts as a speaker, writer, intuitive, coach and mentor.

Bernette's work is aligned with her goal of helping women get and keep their mojo.

She does this as a holistic and intuitive mindset coach with a focus on creating more wellness and wealth for an epic life for herself and other midlife women.

She's published more than a dozen books and had two plays produced, with most works for or featuring sheroes. Bernette also helps aspiring and new authors with self-publishing and public-speaking through her company, Mount Hope Media.

Bernette lives in the Atlanta, Georgia area and is a wife and mother who loves the theater, movies, and coffee.

Links:

Main Website: BernetteSherman.com
Podcast Website: ThatSheroLife.com
Instagram @IAmBernette
Tiktok @IAmBernette
Facebook @IAmBernetteSherman
YouTube @IAmBernette

References

1. Fumero A, Peñate W, Oyanadel C, Porter B. The Effectiveness of Mindfulness-Based Interventions on Anxiety Disorders. A Systematic Meta-Review. European Journal of Investigation in Health, Psychology and Education. 2020; 10(3):704-719. https://doi.org/10.3390/ejihpe10030052

2. Betts JA, Chowdhury EA, Gonzalez JT, Richardson JD, Tsintzas K, Thompson D. Is breakfast the most important meal of the day? Proc Nutr Soc. 2016 Nov;75(4):464-474. doi: 10.1017/S002966 5116000318. Epub 2016 Jun 13. PMID: 27292940.

3. Centers for Disease Control and Prevention. All About Your A1C. 2022 Sep 30. https://www.cdc.gov/diabetes/managing/managing-blood-sugar/a1c.html

4. Centers for Disease Control and Prevention. Antidepressant Use Among Adults: United States, 2015-2018. 2020 Sep. https://www.cdc.gov/nchs/products/databriefs/db377.htm

5. Centers for Disease Control and Prevention. Insulin Resistance and Diabetes. 2022 Jun 20. https://www.cdc.gov/diabetes/basics/insulin-resistance.html

6. Cleveland Clinic. GLP-1 Agonists. Last Reviewed July 3, 2023. https://my.clevelandclinic.org/health/treatments/13901-glp-1-agonists

7. Galioto R, Spitznagel MB. The Effects of Breakfast and Breakfast Composition on Cognition in Adults. Adv Nutr. 2016 May 16;7(3):576S-89S. doi: 10.3945/an.115.010231. PMID: 27184286; PMCID:

PMC4863263.

8. Jakubowicz D, Wainstein J, Tsameret S, Landau Z. Role of High Energy Breakfast "Big Breakfast Diet" in Clock Gene Regulation of Postprandial Hyperglycemia and Weight Loss in Type 2 Diabetes. Nutrients. 2021 May 5;13(5):1558. doi: 10.3390/nu13051558. PMID: 34063109; PMCID: PMC8148179.

9. Jakubowicz D, Barnea M, Wainstein J, Froy O. High caloric intake at breakfast vs. dinner differentially influences weight loss of overweight and obese women. Obesity (Silver Spring). 2013 Dec;21(12):2504-12. doi: 10.1002/oby.20460. Epub 2013 Jul 2. PMID: 23512957.

10. Kelly, K.P, McGuinness O.P., Buchowski, M., Hughey, J.J., Chen, H., Powers, J., Page, T., & Johnson C.H. (2020). Eating breakfast and avoiding late-evening snacking sustains lipid oxidation. PLoS Biol. 18(2): e3000622. https://doi.org/10.1371%2Fjour

nal.pbio.3000622 https://www.ncbi.nlm.ni
h.gov/pmc/articles/PMC7046182/

11. Lopes-Minguez, J.,Gómez-Abellán, P., &
Garaulet, M. (2019). Timing of Breakfast,
Lunch, and Dinner. Effects on Obesity and
Metabolic Risk. Nutrients. 11(11): 2624. ht
tps://doi.org/10.3390%2Fnu11112624

12. Mamerow MM, Mettler JA, English
KL, Casperson SL, Arentson-Lantz E,
Sheffield-Moore M, Layman DK, Pad-
don-Jones D. Dietary protein distribution
positively influences 24-h muscle protein
synthesis in healthy adults. J Nutr. 2014
Jun;144(6):876-80. doi: 10.3945/jn.113.185
280. Epub 2014 Jan 29. PMID: 24477298;
PMCID: PMC4018950.

13. Reutrakul S, Hood MM, Crowley SJ,
Morgan MK, Teodori M, Knutson KL.
The relationship between breakfast skip-
ping, chronotype, and glycemic control
in type 2 diabetes. Chronobiol Int. 2014
Feb;31(1):64-71. doi: 10.3109/07420528.2

013.821614. Epub 2013 Oct 4. PMID: 24094031.

14. Sievert K, Hussain SM, Page MJ, Wang Y, Hughes HJ, Malek M, Cicuttini FM. Effect of breakfast on weight and energy intake: systematic review and meta-analysis of randomised controlled trials. BMJ. 2019 Jan 30;364:l42. doi: 10.1136/bmj.l42. PMID: 30700403; PMCID: PMC6352874.

15. Sleep Foundation. 2024 Mar 1. Chronotypes: Definition, Types, & Effect on Sleep. https://www.sleepfoundation.org/how-sleep-works/chronotypes

16. Smith HA, Betts JA. Nutrient timing and metabolic regulation. J Physiol. 2022 Mar;600(6):1299-1312. doi: 10.1113/JP280756. Epub 2022 Jan 31. PMID: 35038774; PMCID: PMC9305539.

17. Van der Kolk B. The Body Keeps the Score. Penguin Books. ISBN: 978-0-14-312774-1. 2015.

18. Vignola N. Rewire. Harper Collins. ISBN: 978-0-06-334979-7. 2024.

19. Weid, H. Number of steps per day more important than step intensity. National Institutes of Health. 2020 Mar. https://www.nih.gov/news-events/nih-research-matters/number-steps-day-more-important-step-intensity

20. Xiao Q, Garaulet M, Scheer FAJL. Meal timing and obesity: interactions with macronutrient intake and chronotype. Int J Obes (Lond). 2019 Sep;43(9):1701-1711. doi: 10.1038/s41366-018-0284-x. Epub 2019 Jan 31. PMID: 30705391; PMCID: PMC6669101.

Made in the USA
Columbia, SC
23 September 2024